PLANNING FOR LONG-TERM USE OF BIOMEDICAL DATA

PROCEEDINGS OF A WORKSHOP

Linda Casola, *Rapporteur*

Board on Mathematical Sciences and Analytics

Committee on Applied and Theoretical Statistics

Computer Science and Telecommunications Board

Division on Engineering and Physical Sciences

Board on Life Sciences
Division on Earth and Life Studies

Board on Research Data and Information
Policy and Global Affairs

The National Academies of
SCIENCES · ENGINEERING · MEDICINE

THE NATIONAL ACADEMIES PRESS
Washington, DC
www.nap.edu

THE NATIONAL ACADEMIES PRESS 500 Fifth Street, NW Washington, DC 20001

This activity was supported by Contract No. HHSN263002 with the National Institutes of Health. Any opinions, findings, conclusions, or recommendations expressed in this publication do not necessarily reflect the views of any organization or agency that provided support for the project.

International Standard Book Number-13: 978-0-309-67275-7
International Standard Book Number-10: 0-309-67275-9
Digital Object Identifier: https://doi.org/10.17226/25707

Additional copies of this publication are available from the National Academies Press, 500 Fifth Street, NW, Keck 360, Washington, DC 20001; (800) 624-6242 or (202) 334-3313; http://www.nap.edu.

Copyright 2020 by the National Academy of Sciences. All rights reserved.

Printed in the United States of America

Suggested citation: National Academies of Sciences, Engineering, and Medicine. 2020. *Planning for Long-Term Use of Biomedical Data: Proceedings of a Workshop.* Washington, DC: The National Academies Press. https://doi.org/10.17226/25707.

The National Academies of
SCIENCES · ENGINEERING · MEDICINE

The **National Academy of Sciences** was established in 1863 by an Act of Congress, signed by President Lincoln, as a private, nongovernmental institution to advise the nation on issues related to science and technology. Members are elected by their peers for outstanding contributions to research. Dr. Marcia McNutt is president.

The **National Academy of Engineering** was established in 1964 under the charter of the National Academy of Sciences to bring the practices of engineering to advising the nation. Members are elected by their peers for extraordinary contributions to engineering. Dr. John L. Anderson is president.

The **National Academy of Medicine** (formerly the Institute of Medicine) was established in 1970 under the charter of the National Academy of Sciences to advise the nation on medical and health issues. Members are elected by their peers for distinguished contributions to medicine and health. Dr. Victor J. Dzau is president.

The three Academies work together as the **National Academies of Sciences, Engineering, and Medicine** to provide independent, objective analysis and advice to the nation and conduct other activities to solve complex problems and inform public policy decisions. The National Academies also encourage education and research, recognize outstanding contributions to knowledge, and increase public understanding in matters of science, engineering, and medicine.

Learn more about the National Academies of Sciences, Engineering, and Medicine at **www.nationalacademies.org**.

The National Academies of
SCIENCES • ENGINEERING • MEDICINE

Consensus Study Reports published by the National Academies of Sciences, Engineering, and Medicine document the evidence-based consensus on the study's statement of task by an authoring committee of experts. Reports typically include findings, conclusions, and recommendations based on information gathered by the committee and the committee's deliberations. Each report has been subjected to a rigorous and independent peer-review process and it represents the position of the National Academies on the statement of task.

Proceedings published by the National Academies of Sciences, Engineering, and Medicine chronicle the presentations and discussions at a workshop, symposium, or other event convened by the National Academies. The statements and opinions contained in proceedings are those of the participants and are not endorsed by other participants, the planning committee, or the National Academies.

For information about other products and activities of the National Academies, please visit www.nationalacademies.org/about/whatwedo.

COMMITTEE ON THE WORKSHOP ON FORECASTING COSTS FOR PRESERVING AND PROMOTING ACCESS TO BIOMEDICAL DATA

DAVID S.C. CHU, Institute for Defense Analyses, *Chair*
ILKAY ALTINTAS, University of California, San Diego
G. SAYEED CHOUDHURY, Johns Hopkins University
MARGARET LEVENSTEIN, University of Michigan
CLIFFORD A. LYNCH, Coalition for Networked Information
DAVID MAIER, Portland State University
CHARLES F. MANSKI, NAS,[1] Northwestern University
MARYANN MARTONE, University of California, San Diego
ALEXA T. McCRAY, NAM,[2] Harvard Medical School
MICHELLE MEYER, Geisinger
WILLIAM W. STEAD, NAM, Vanderbilt University Medical Center
LARS VILHUBER, Cornell University

Staff

TYLER KLOEFKORN, Program Officer, Board on Mathematical Sciences and Analytics, *Workshop Director*
SAMMANTHA L. MAGSINO, Senior Program Officer, Board on Earth Sciences and Resources, *Study Director*
SELAM ARAIA, Senior Program Assistant, Board on Mathematical Sciences and Analytics
LINDA CASOLA, Associate Program Officer, Board on Mathematical Sciences and Analytics
CHRISTOPHER FU, Research Associate, Board on Mathematical Sciences and Analytics
ADRIANNA HARGROVE, Financial Manager
MICHELLE SCHWALBE, Director, Board on Mathematical Sciences and Analytics
LINDA WALKER, Program Coordinator, Board on Physics and Astronomy

---

[1] Member, National Academy of Sciences.
[2] Member, National Academy of Medicine.

BOARD ON MATHEMATICAL SCIENCES AND ANALYTICS

MARK L. GREEN, University of California, Los Angeles, *Chair*
HÉLÈNE BARCELO, Mathematical Sciences Research Institute
JOHN R. BIRGE, NAE,[1] University of Chicago
W. PETER CHERRY, NAE, Independent Consultant
DAVID S.C. CHU, Institute for Defense Analyses
RONALD R. COIFMAN, NAS,[2] Yale University
JAMES (JIM) CURRY, University of Colorado Boulder
SHAWNDRA HILL, Microsoft Research
LYDIA KAVRAKI, NAM,[3] Rice University
TAMARA KOLDA, Sandia National Laboratories
JOSEPH A. LANGSAM, University of Maryland, College Park
DAVID MAIER, Portland State University
LOIS CURFMAN McINNES, Argonne National Laboratory
JILL PIPHER, Brown University
ELIZABETH A. THOMPSON, NAS, University of Washington
CLAIRE TOMLIN, NAE, University of California, Berkeley
LANCE WALLER, Emory University
KAREN E. WILLCOX, University of Texas, Austin

Staff

MICHELLE SCHWALBE, Director
SELAM ARAIA, Senior Program Assistant
LINDA CASOLA, Associate Program Officer
CHRISTOPHER FU, Research Associate (until August 2019)
ADRIANNA HARGROVE, Finance Business Partner
TYLER KLOEFKORN, Program Officer

---

[1] Member, National Academy of Engineering.
[2] Member, National Academy of Sciences.
[3] Member, National Academy of Medicine.

COMMITTEE ON APPLIED AND THEORETICAL STATISTICS

ALFRED O. HERO III, University of Michigan, *Chair*
ALICIA CARRIQUIRY, NAM,[1] Iowa State University
RONG CHEN, Rutgers University, The State University of New Jersey
MICHAEL J. DANIELS, University of Florida
KATHERINE BENNETT ENSOR, Rice University
AMY H. HERRING, Duke University
TIM HESTERBERG, Google, Inc.
NICHOLAS J. HORTON, Amherst College
DAVID MADIGAN, Columbia University
XIAO-LI MENG, Harvard University
JOSÉ M.F. MOURA, NAE,[2] Carnegie Mellon University
RAQUEL PRADO, University of California, Santa Cruz
NANCY M. REID, NAS,[3] University of Toronto
CYNTHIA RUDIN, Duke University
AARTI SINGH, Carnegie Mellon University
ALYSON G. WILSON, North Carolina State University

Staff

TYLER KLOEFKORN, Director
SELAM ARAIA, Senior Program Assistant
LINDA CASOLA, Associate Program Officer
CHRISTOPHER FU, Research Associate (until August 2019)
ADRIANNA HARGROVE, Financial Manager

---

[1] Member, National Academy of Medicine.
[2] Member, National Academy of Engineering.
[3] Member, National Academy of Sciences.

COMPUTER SCIENCE AND TELECOMMUNICATIONS BOARD

FARNAM JAHANIAN, Carnegie Mellon University, *Chair*
STEVEN M. BELLOVIN, NAE,[1] Columbia University
DAVID CULLER, NAE, University of California, Berkeley
EDWARD FRANK, NAE, Cloud Parity, Inc.
LAURA HAAS, NAE, University of Massachusetts Amherst
ERIC HORVITZ, NAE, Microsoft Corporation
BETH MYNATT, Georgia Institute of Technology
CRAIG PARTRIDGE, Colorado State University
DANIELA RUS, NAE, Massachusetts Institute of Technology
FRED B. SCHNEIDER, NAE, Cornell University
MARGO SELTZER, University of British Columbia
MOSHE VARDI, NAS[2]/NAE, Rice University

Staff

JON EISENBERG, Senior Board Director
SHENAE BRADLEY, Administrative Assistant
RENEE HAWKINS, Financial and Administrative Manager
LYNETTE I. MILLETT, Associate Director
KATIRIA ORTIZ, Associate Program Officer

---

[1] Member, National Academy of Engineering.
[2] Member, National Academy of Sciences.

BOARD ON LIFE SCIENCES

JAMES P. COLLINS, Arizona State University, *Chair*
A. ALONSO AGUIRRE, George Mason University
ENRIQUETA C. BOND, NAM,[1] Burroughs Wellcome Fund
DOMINIQUE BROSSARD, University of Wisconsin–Madison
ROGER D. CONE, NAS[2]/NAM, University of Michigan
NANCY D. CONNELL, Johns Hopkins Center for Health Security
SEAN M. DECATUR, Kenyon College
JOSEPH R. ECKER, NAS, Howard Hughes Medical Institute
SCOTT V. EDWARDS, NAS, Harvard University
GERALD L. EPSTEIN, National Defense University
ROBERT J. FULL, University of California, Berkeley
ELIZABETH HEITMAN, University of Texas Southwestern Medical Center
MARY E. MAXON, Lawrence Berkeley National Laboratory
ROBERT NEWMAN, Independent Consultant
STEPHEN J. O'BRIEN, NAS, Nova Southeastern University
CLAIRE POMEROY, NAM, The Albert and Mary Lasker Foundation
MARY E. POWER, NAS, University of California, Berkeley
SUSAN RUNDELL SINGER, Rollins College
LANA SKIRBOLL, Sanofi
DAVID R. WALT, NAE[3]/NAM, Harvard Medical School

Staff

FRAN SHARPLES, Director
LIDA ANESTIDOU, Senior Program Officer
KATHERINE BOWMAN, Senior Program Officer
JESSICA DE MOUY, Senior Program Assistant
ANDREA HODGSON, Program Officer
JO HUSBANDS, Scholar/Senior Project Director
KEEGAN SAWYER, Senior Program Officer
AUDREY THEVENON, Program Officer
KOSSANA YOUNG, Senior Program Assistant

---

[1] Member, National Academy of Medicine.
[2] Member, National Academy of Sciences.
[3] Member, National Academy of Engineering.

BOARD ON RESEARCH DATA AND INFORMATION

ALEXA T. MCCRAY, NAM,[1] Harvard Medical School, *Chair*
AMY BRAND, Massachusetts Institute of Technology Press
STUART FELDMAN, Schmidt Futures
SALMAN HABIB, Argonne National Laboratory
JAMES HENDLER, Rensselaer Polytechnic Institute
ELLIOT E. MAXWELL, e-Maxwell and Associates
BAREND MONS, Leiden University Medical Centre
SARAH NUSSER, Iowa State University
MICHAEL STEBBINS, Science Advisors, LLC

Staff

GEORGE STRAWN, Director
ESTER SZTEIN, Deputy Director
TOM ARRISON, Program Director
ADRIANA COUREMBIS, Financial Officer
REGINALD HAYES, Senior Program Assistant
EMI KAMEYAMA, Associate Program Officer

---

[1] Member, National Academy of Medicine.

Acknowledgment of Reviewers

This Proceedings of a Workshop was reviewed in draft form by individuals chosen for their diverse perspectives and technical expertise. The purpose of this independent review is to provide candid and critical comments that will assist the National Academies of Sciences, Engineering, and Medicine in making each published proceedings as sound as possible and to ensure that it meets the institutional standards for quality, objectivity, evidence, and responsiveness to the charge. The review comments and draft manuscript remain confidential to protect the integrity of the process.

We thank the following individuals for their review of this proceedings: Warren Kibbe, Duke University, and Michelle Meyer, Geisinger. We also thank staff member Scott Weidman for reading and providing helpful comments on the manuscript.

Although the reviewers listed above provided many constructive comments and suggestions, they were not asked to endorse the content of the proceedings nor did they see the final draft before its release. The review of this proceedings was overseen by Bradford H. Gray, NAM,[1] The Urban Institute (retired). He was responsible for making certain that an independent examination of this proceedings was carried out in accordance with the standards of the National Academies and that all review comments were carefully considered. Responsibility for the final content rests entirely with the rapporteur and the National Academies.

---

[1] Member, National Academy of Medicine.

Contents

1 INTRODUCTION 1
　Workshop Overview, 1
　Opening Remarks, 3

2 DATA SHARING AND DATA PRESERVATION 7
　The Burdens and Benefits of "Long-Tail" Data Sharing, 7
　Panel Discussion: Researchers' Perspectives on Managing Risks
　　and Forecasting Costs for Long-Term Data Preservation, 13

3 DATA RISKS AND COSTS 20
　Panel Discussion: Addressing Data Risks and Their Costs, 20
　Summaries of Small-Group Discussions, 26

4 TOOLS AND PRACTICES FOR RISK MANAGEMENT,
　DATA PRESERVATION, AND ACCESSING DECISIONS 29
　Data—What's It Going to Cost and What's in It for Me?, 29
　Precisely Practicing Medicine from 700 Trillion Points of Data, 32

5 LIFETIME DATA COSTS 38
　Panel Discussion: Incentives, Mechanisms, and Practices
　　for Improved Awareness of Cost Consequences in
　　Data Decisions, 38
　Summaries of Small-Group Discussions, 47

6	REFLECTIONS AND NEXT STEPS Panel Discussion: Researchers' Perspectives on Next Steps, 50 Themes and Opportunities, 54	50

REFERENCES 59

APPENDIXES

A	Workshop Agenda	63
B	Biographical Sketches of Committee	67
C	Registered In-Person Workshop Participants	76

1

Introduction

WORKSHOP OVERVIEW

Biomedical research data sets are becoming larger and more complex, and computing capabilities are expanding to enable transformative scientific results. The National Institutes of Health's (NIH's) National Library of Medicine (NLM) has the unique role of ensuring that biomedical research data are findable, accessible, interoperable, and reusable in an ethical manner. Tools that forecast the costs of long-term data preservation could be useful as the cost to curate and manage these data in meaningful ways continues to increase, as could stewardship to assess and maintain data that have future value.

The National Academies of Sciences, Engineering, and Medicine's Board on Mathematical Sciences and Analytics (in cooperation with the Computer Science and Telecommunications Board, the Board on Life Sciences, and the Board on Research Data and Information) was charged by NLM to undertake a consensus study. The Committee on Forecasting Costs for Preserving, Archiving, and Promoting Access to Biomedical Data was tasked with developing and demonstrating a framework for forecasting long-term costs for preserving, archiving, and accessing biomedical data and estimating future potential benefits to research (see Box 1.1 for the committee's statement of task). To gather insight and information from the community on these issues, the committee convened a workshop on July 11–12, 2019, at the National Academy of Sciences building in Washington, DC (see Appendix A for the workshop agenda). The committee's role was limited to organizing the workshop (see Appendix B for

1

biographies of the committee members). Approximately 75 participants attended the workshop (see Appendix C), with additional participation online.

This proceedings is a factual summary of what occurred at the workshop. The views contained in this proceedings are those of the individual workshop participants and do not necessarily represent the views of the participants as a whole, the committee, or the National Academies of Sciences, Engineering, and Medicine.

BOX 1.1
Statement of Task

A National Academies of Sciences, Engineering, and Medicine–appointed ad hoc committee will develop and demonstrate a framework for forecasting long-term costs for preserving, archiving, and accessing various types of biomedical data and estimating potential future benefits to research. In so doing, the committee will examine and evaluate the following considerations:
- Economic factors to be considered when examining the life-cycle cost for data sets (e.g., data acquisition, preservation, and dissemination);
- Cost consequences for various practices in accessioning and de-accessioning data sets;
- Economic factors to be considered in designating data sets as high value;
- Assumptions built in to the data collection and/or modeling processes;
- Anticipated technological disruptors and future developments in data science in a 5- to 10-year horizon; and
- Critical factors for successful adoption of data forecasting approaches by research and program management staff.

The committee will provide two case studies illustrating application of the framework to different biomedical contexts relevant to the National Library of Medicine's data resources. Relevant life-cycle costs will be delineated, as well as the assumptions underlying the models. To the extent practicable, the committee will identify strategies to communicate results and gain acceptance of the applicability of these models.

As part of its information gathering, the committee will plan and organize a 2-day workshop to gather input on the following topics:
- Tools and practices that NLM could use to help researchers and funders better integrate risk management practices and considerations into data preservation, archiving, and accessing decisions;
- Methods to encourage NIH-funded researchers to consider, update, and track lifetime data costs (e.g., through data management plans and project renewals, or other interactions with the NIH); and
- Burdens on the academic researchers and industry staff to implement these tools, methods, and practices.

OPENING REMARKS

David Chu, Institute for Defense Analyses
Patricia Flatley Brennan, National Library of Medicine

David Chu, Institute for Defense Analyses, explained that workshop participants would have the opportunity to discuss (1) tools and practices that NLM could use to help researchers and funders better integrate risk management practices and considerations into data preservation, archiving, and accessing decisions; (2) methods to encourage NIH-funded researchers to consider, update, and track lifetime data costs; and (3) burdens on the academic researchers and industry staff to implement these tools, methods, and practices. To frame these discussions, he posed key questions about the decision making involved in forecasting costs: What is being acquired, and/or what specific activity is being supported? What are the parameters for estimating cost, and how will they change over time? What are the distributions that characterize these parameters? Who is performing the activities, and what incentives might affect their behaviors?

Chu noted that NLM serves as an important resource for biomedical discovery through its substantial data and information resources. Patricia Flatley Brennan, NLM, stated that 5 million people interact with NIH's data repositories, resources, data sets, and literature each day; these activities benefit clinicians, patients, researchers, industry, government agencies, and pharmaceutical companies. She expressed her hope that increased data sharing in coordination with expertise and tools from the mathematical sciences and computational sciences communities will lead to novel discoveries in human health.

With 27 research institutes and centers, NIH is the world's largest funder of biomedical research. However, Brennan continued, having 27 different approaches to the same problem creates challenges. Instead of each institute having its own data management strategy and plans, Brennan explained that NIH's goal is to adopt enterprise-level solutions that will garner the greatest return on its research investments. As a result, NIH could become an "ecosphere of discovery" (i.e., a knowledge and discovery platform), with aspects of the research process connected across time (see Figure 1.1).

She explained that protocols, literature, clinical data, codes, and pathways are all research products that need to be curated, preserved, and reused. Thus, it is important to consider how to best preserve data with a high level of integrity over the long term—data generated in the past and present should be available to use for future scientific discoveries, she asserted. The role of the researcher is evolving, too. Instead of serving only as data generators, researchers will become data contributors,

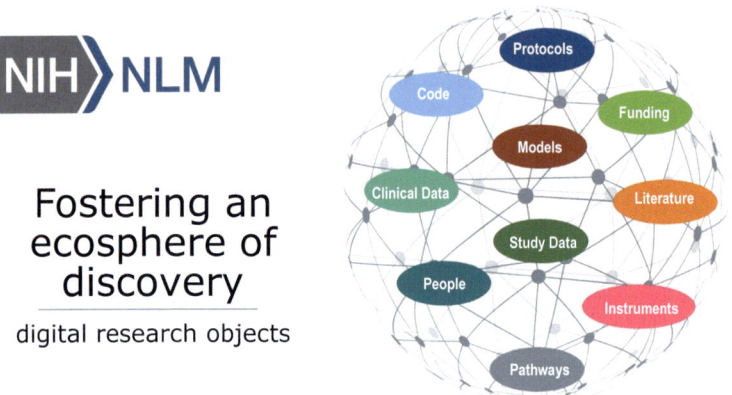

FIGURE 1.1 Fostering an ecosphere of discovery with digital research products. SOURCE: Patricia Flatley Brennan, National Library of Medicine, presentation to the workshop, July 11, 2019.

data users, data miners, data analysts, and data scientists. She noted that this change corresponds to a shift in the research process from the use of experimental and observational models to data-driven discovery.

Brennan said that NIH actively encourages the use of open access data repositories[1] for data generated throughout the course of the research process and oversees several data storage activities. PubMed Central,[2] which currently hosts more than 5 million articles and adds between 5,000 and 7,000 data sets each month, is best suited for investigator-curated data sets up to 2 GB. These data sets receive Digital Object Identifiers and can be attached to PubMed Central's full-text articles. To manage larger data sets, NIH established partnerships with Dryad[3] and FigShare.[4] These repositories are best suited for data sets up to 20 GB. PubMed citations direct researchers to specific FigShare data sets with unique identifiers; however, FigShare lacks the appropriate protections to store human data. For high-priority data sets in the terabyte range, NIH manages its own repositories. NIH has a scientific data enterprise strategy initiative (Science and Technology Research Infrastructure for Discovery,

---

[1] For more information about NIH's initiatives, see https://www.nlm.nih.gov/NIHbmic/nih_data_sharing_repositories.html, accessed August 2, 2019.

[2] For more information on PubMed Central, see https://www.ncbi.nlm.nih.gov/pmc, accessed October 8, 2019.

[3] For more information on Dryad, see https://datadryad.org/stash, accessed October 8, 2019.

[4] For more information on FigShare, see figshare.com, accessed October 8, 2019.

Experimentation, and Sustainability [STRIDES][5]) to repurpose commercial cloud space and make data sets available to the general public and to scientists around the world, as well as via controlled access with a token-based identity management system. In July 2019, NIH's National Center for Biotechnology Information uploaded 5 PB of a nonhuman sequence read archive into the cloud system, which will be available via Google Cloud and Amazon Web Services for public access.

Brennan explained that each year, NIH spends $30 billion to generate data, more than $1 billion to manage NIH data in various repositories, and approximately $250 million to support data repositories in postsecondary institutions.[6] She noted that there are political, sociological, and scientific questions embedded in decisions about the allocation of funds toward data sustainability in particular, and there are substantial hidden costs in data management. She emphasized that NIH needs tools to understand how much it is spending and how to spend more wisely (see Figure 1.2).

With an enterprise data management strategy, investigators could use these tools to plan for research challenges and the costs associated with future data sets; this would ensure that the most useful data are preserved and that research budgets for individual investigators are maintained, Brennan said. The forecasting framework that the National Academies' committee will develop over the course of its study could be used by researchers, program officers, and funders alike, she continued. She hoped that this workshop would help illuminate the incentives and barriers to depositing data, the obstacles to subsequent use of data, and the potential markets for the reuse of data.

---

[5] For more information about the Science and Technology Research Infrastructure for Discovery, Experimentation, and Sustainability initiative, see https://datascience.nih.gov/strides, accessed October 8, 2019.

[6] In other words, NIH spends approximately 3 percent on data management and less than 1 percent to support data management and repositories in postsecondary institutions. The NIH released its Data Management and Sharing Plan proposal in November 2019; see https://www.federalregister.gov/documents/2019/11/08/2019-24529/request-for-public-comments-on-a-draft-nih-policy-for-data-management-and-sharing-and-supplemental.

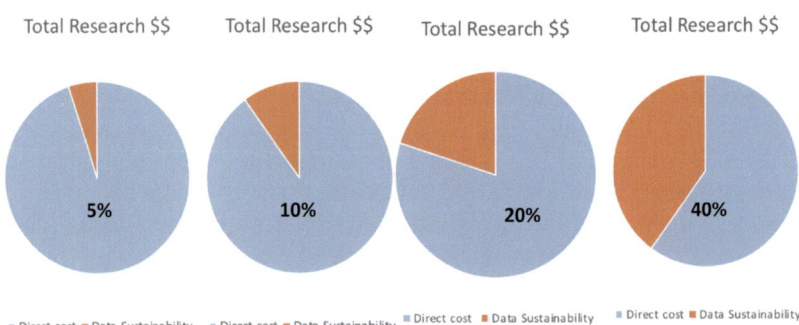

FIGURE 1.2 Possible future investment strategies for data sustainability.
SOURCE: Patricia Flatley Brennan, National Library of Medicine, presentation to the workshop, July 11, 2019.

2

Data Sharing and Data Preservation

THE BURDENS AND BENEFITS OF "LONG-TAIL" DATA SHARING

Adam Ferguson, University of California, San Francisco

Adam Ferguson, University of California, San Francisco, explained that injuries to the central nervous system (CNS) are incredibly complex, in part because the human brain has 100 trillion synapses and the spinal cord has hundreds of billions of synapses. This complexity creates a data science problem with implications for public health. Traumatic brain injuries (TBIs) cost $400 billion annually worldwide, and spinal cord injuries (SCIs) cost $40 billion annually in the United States alone. Magnifying the problem is the absence of any U.S. Food and Drug Administration–approved therapies for TBIs or SCIs alongside the abundance of tiny measures of biofunction related to TBIs and SCIs. Ferguson asserted that sharing data and making them interoperable is the best strategy to better understand these complex disorders.

Ferguson described the bottleneck that is created when researchers perform data entry and curation on enormous amounts of heterogeneous raw data. He asserted that databases are not typically equipped to handle volume, velocity, and variety of data, the last of which is particularly relevant in the study of CNS injuries. He explained that relatively little organized big data exist throughout biomedicine. Most data fall in the long tail of the distribution, where there are modestly sized data sets and many heterogeneous data sets.

Ferguson said that published literature contains approximately 15 percent of data, which means that approximately 85 percent of data collected worldwide for biomedical research is unpublished, "dark" data. He estimated that more than $200 billion of the $240 billion worldwide annual biomedical research budget is wasted on data that are inaccessible (see Macleod et al., 2014). Furthermore, because all of the published biomedical literature contains only 15 percent of the total data collected, published research represents a biased sample of the full range of biomedical data available (see Ioannidis, 2015). Ferguson described this as a systemic problem within scientific publications, which *summarize* data instead of *provide* data. Researchers spend most of their time creating protocols, and information can be lost during the process of developing a brief high-impact paper (see Figure 2.1). This "ancient data-sharing technology" for biomedical research should be replaced with modern data repositories, he asserted.

Ferguson described an initiative to create a multispecies data repository called VISION-SCI, which contains approximately 60 million data points from 4,000 rats and mice with SCIs. These data are comingled with deidentified human medical records. This effort began with a $1 million grant for data curation but enabled access to nearly $70 million of prior research investment and data collection from the National Institutes of Health (NIH). He added that post-data collection cleaning and curation (the need for which is realized at the point of data sharing) typically requires 15–20 percent of a researcher's total budget.

The SCI Open Data Commons initiative[1] is another path forward in the field—it hosts a web portal that allows people to access VISION-SCI and to contribute and manage their own data. This initiative has expanded with the development of the TBI Open Data Commons[2] and the Veterans Affairs Gordon Mansfield SCI Consortium,[3] the latter of which is focused on translational SCI stem cell therapies. Ferguson also described Transforming Research and Clinical Knowledge (TRACK)-TBI[4] and TRACK-SCI, which are large-scale clinical observation studies designed to generate high-quality clinical data. In July 2019, TRACK-TBI had 3,500 patients enrolled from 18 U.S. Level-1 trauma centers. He pointed out that all of these initiatives are guided by the FAIR (findable, accessible, interoperable, reusable) principles for data stewardship—biomedical research data

---

[1] For more information about the SCI Open Data Commons, see https://scicrunch.org/odc-sci, accessed August 2, 2019.

[2] For more information about the TBI Open Data Commons, see http://odc-tbi.org, accessed August 2, 2019.

[3] For more information about the Veterans Affairs Gordon Mansfield SCI Consortium, see http://grantome.com/grant/NIH/I50-RX001706-01, accessed October 8, 2019.

[4] For more information about TRACK-TBI, see https://tracktbi.ucsf.edu/transforming-research-and-clinical-knowledge-tbi, accessed October 8, 2019.

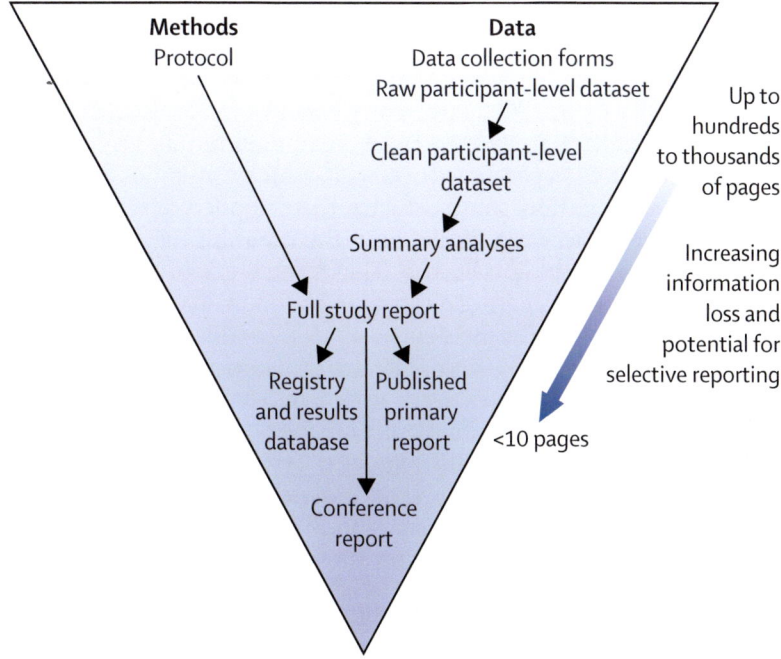

FIGURE 2.1 The process of scientific publication. SOURCE: Republished with permission of *The Lancet*, from A.-W. Chan, et al., Increasing value and reducing waste: Addressing inaccessible research, *The Lancet* 383:9913, 2014; permission conveyed through Copyright Clearance Center, Inc.

should be *findable* (i.e., data and metadata are "uniquely and persistently identifiable" as well as human and machine readable), *accessible* (i.e., data are "reachable" by humans and machines "using standard formats and protocols"), *interoperable* (i.e., "data are machine readable and annotated with resolvable vocabularies and ontologies," which is particularly challenging), and *reusable* (i.e., data are harmonized with data from other contributors) (Wilkinson et al., 2016). Following these guidelines elevates biomedical data from raw material to primary work products, he explained.

The SCI community was an early adopter of the FAIR principles, hosting a workshop in 2016 on FAIR data sharing,[5] a workshop in 2017 on the policy needed to execute FAIR data sharing via an open data commons,[6]

---

[5] For more information, see https://www.ninds.nih.gov/News-Events/Events-Proceedings/Events/Spinal-Cord-Injury-Preclinical-Data-Workshop-Developing-FAIR, accessed September 12, 2019.

[6] For more information, see https://www.sfn.org/Meetings/Neuroscience-2017, accessed September 12, 2019.

and a community hackathon in 2018,[7] during which participants uploaded their data to the SCI Open Data Commons. He emphasized that digital development is not possible without support from the research community. For example, the SCI community constructed a private space to make data accessible. A researcher can upload data to this private space and deposit them in the open data commons, which comingles data across laboratories. Data citation standards are then applied via SciCrunch,[8] Digital Object Identifiers are issued, and the data are released under a creative commons attribution license. This framework provides a single place in which SCI researchers can organize and publish their data as well as receive primary credit for the data as a work product.

Many opportunities arise once data are organized within this framework. For example, Ferguson's team uses Syndromic Data Integration, which suggests that any individual outcome measure is but one potential window into the underlying syndrome of a CNS injury. His team's primary objective is to understand how an individual compares to a group of individuals on particular variables. With the help of machine learning, individuals can be clustered based on their multidimensional location within the syndromic space. This level of understanding places a renewed emphasis on precision and reproducibility, he continued.

Ferguson concluded his presentation by sharing an anecdote about researcher Jessica Nielson, University of Minnesota, who made use of the 1994–1996 Multicenter Animal SCI Study (MASCIS), which was a blinded randomized multidrug multicenter clinical trial in rats. The data from this study were dispersed across shelves at seven U.S. laboratories after the hypothesis was disproven. Nielson collected these data from binders, scanned them into PDFs, and used machine learning tools to understand why the trial failed. She learned that despite having the same biomechanical injuries, two groups in the trial had dramatically different locomotor outcomes. Animals with high blood pressure on the operating table had poor long-term prognoses. She realized that blood pressure during SCI surgery was the predictor of long-term locomotor recovery, not medication (Nielson et al., 2015). Although researchers have long focused on how to avoid low blood pressure in humans in the operating room, this evidence could now prompt clinical research studies on the effects of high blood pressure in the operating room. Maryann Martone, University of California, San Diego, wondered what prompted Nielson to collect the records from MASCIS since animal records are generally not considered

---

[7] For more information, see https://scicrunch.org/odc-sci/about/blog/1481, accessed September 12, 2019.
[8] For more information about SciCrunch, see https://scicrunch.org, accessed August 2, 2019.

to be "data." Ferguson responded that MASCIS was organized similar to a randomized control trial, with standardized forms and binders at all seven sites. As an SCI researcher, Nielson thought that there was value in animal research when treated like human clinical data. Ferguson asserted that generating new knowledge from old data reduces the number of animals used in future clinical trials (see Neff, 2018; Chakradhar, 2017) and advances data-driven scientific discovery.

David Chu, Institute for Defense Analyses, noted the value of sample design when the cost to collect all data points is too high. He pointed out that nonstatistically significant results are often crucial for scientific understanding, and he wondered whether researchers should sample dark data instead of trying to preserve all data. Ferguson noted that, with enough data and the application of appropriate machine learning methods, it might be possible to estimate effect sizes. Further, the amount of dark data being collected in biomedicine could be reduced if the community better supported data sharing.

Robert Williams, University of Tennessee Health Science Center, said that the creation of a journal series via Jupyter Lab Notebooks could help address long-tail data issues, although this may increase publication costs for researchers. Ferguson speculated that publications in the future might resemble the Internet—one could click to source data from links within a web-based version of an article. Patricia Flatley Brennan, National Library of Medicine (NLM), noted that the need for investigator interpretation of data will always exist; it is an investigator's responsibility to share his or her perspective on data, especially when interim artifacts (e.g., preprints, models, and protocols) could be reconstituted by another investigator. Sharing data via publications is not sustainable because there may be multiple data resources linked to one publication or multiple publications linked to a single data resource. She explained that it is critical to understand future relationships among publication, accountability, knowledge building, and the roles that archival data can play.

William Stead, Vanderbilt University Medical Center, asked how Ferguson's approaches to data sharing could reduce costs over time and increase sustainability. Ferguson said that data are more likely to be reused if they are made digital earlier in the process and if stakeholders have direct input into the study design. Jessie Tenenbaum, Duke University and the North Carolina Department of Health and Human Services, described her desire to "make data a first class citizen" (by prioritizing curation and annotation early in the process) and wondered if doing so is practical. Ferguson agreed that data should be a "first class citizen" and said that the adoption of standards (similar to peer review) is the key. Ilkay Altintas, University of California, San Diego, wondered about the potential for machine learning and artificial intelligence to be "disruptors" for data curation, and Ferguson proposed inserting machine learning earlier in the curation process. Altintas predicted that there would be issues due to conflicting curation procedures between private and public archives and wondered how to capture the cost of curation if it is done automatically.

In response to a question about curation costs and associated standards from Alexa McCray, Harvard Medical School, Ferguson said that data curation costs increase when many thousands of variables are present in siloed data systems. He explained that although common data elements may exist in two data sets, interoperability drifts over time as various people begin to recode variables in published papers. Sarah Nusser, Iowa State University, estimated that data curation costs are 20 percent in the fields of astronomy and physics, and any large-scale research operation requires significant preplanning around the collection of information. She wondered how researchers should think, from the front end, about sharing data. Ferguson said that prospective clinical studies have a direct analogy to astronomy and physics in that they include a substantial amount of preplanning and still have high costs. He hopes to use findings from a study of ultra-dark data in the preclinical space to build living common data elements that can be updated more rapidly. An online participant wondered if costs for curation would decrease with the use of new methodologies to collect data. Ferguson expressed his hope that as data become increasingly digital, people will start to drive costs down by doing more curation at the front end of the process.

Ferguson said that the 10–15 percent of an overall project budget being used for curation is an over-time cost as opposed to an upfront cost (i.e., it is not included in the initial funding). Ferguson added that once data are collected and stored in an informatics system, registration requires significant personnel time. Warren Kibbe, Duke University, noted that a transformational cost still exists even with digital data; thus, cleaning data for a second time (and a different purpose) has to be accounted for in the total cost.

Brennan emphasized the need to consider the costs of curation at the point of use. Brad Malin, Vanderbilt University Medical Center, said that these costs are extremely high. For example, NIH's All of Us Research Program[9] is tasked with capturing genomic data, medical records data, and survey data on 1 million Americans; harmonizing these data; and making them accessible to the public. This post-hoc harmonization of electronic medical records data is a multiyear effort, Malin explained. Defining the

---

[9] For more information about the All of Us Research Program, see Allofus.nih.gov, accessed September 25, 2019.

Observational Medical Outcomes Partnership (OMOP)[10] language was relatively simple, but, at times, it has been difficult to translate the data onto a model because many records have incomplete or incorrect data, he continued. Problems also arise when there are differences in measurement techniques. He estimated that millions of dollars of an approximately $100 million budget are being spent to get the data into a usable form. Lars Vilhuber, Cornell University, said that what Malin described could be considered secondary data acquisition (as opposed to curation at the point of use), which results in an additional substantial expense. Philip Bourne, University of Virginia, observed that culture plays a prominent role in any discussion about curation at the point of collection and at the point of use—people have false expectations for the future based on what has happened in the past.

Monica McCormick, University of Delaware Library, asked about the role of the individual university in curation: Where should the tools be developed, and where should the training occur? Ferguson responded that it would be ideal if more university libraries accepted these responsibilities. Vilhuber pointed out that Ferguson's streamlined approach to organize and publish data places more value on the data and thus increases the incentives to share and reuse data. However, if data are protected only by a creative commons attribution license, researchers might not have control over or earn credit for how those data are used in the future. Ferguson noted that a researcher's motivation for sharing data is typically to advance scientific discovery. He added that it is unclear what motives prevent researchers from sharing their data; however, these motives will become clearer if funders begin to enforce data-sharing policies.

PANEL DISCUSSION: RESEARCHERS' PERSPECTIVES ON MANAGING RISKS AND FORECASTING COSTS FOR LONG-TERM DATA PRESERVATION

Margaret Levenstein, University of Michigan, Moderator
Nuno Bandeira, University of California, San Diego
Jessie Tenenbaum, Duke University and the North Carolina Department of Health and Human Services
Georgia (Gina) Tourassi, Oak Ridge National Laboratory
Robert Williams, University of Tennessee Health Science Center

Margaret Levenstein, University of Michigan, moderated a panel discussion among researchers who were asked to share their individual

---

[10] For more information about the Observational Medical Outcomes Partnership, see https://fnih.org/what-we-do/major-completed-programs/omop, accessed December 5, 2019.

perspectives on (1) managing risks and forecasting costs for long-term data preservation, archiving, and accessing decisions, with consideration for different kinds of biomedical data (e.g., clinical data, survey data, imaging data, genomic data) and research endeavors (e.g., collecting new data and leveraging existing data assets); (2) methods to encourage NIH-funded researchers to consider, update, and track lifetime data costs; and (3) challenges for academic researchers and industry staff to implement these tools, methods, and practices. She emphasized that expanding data curation and data-sharing efforts requires cultural change. With the data revolution, the roles of both data users and data producers are changing.

Nuno Bandeira, University of California, San Diego, described his interest in the development of algorithms for interpreting mass spectrometry data in metabolomics, proteomics, and natural products. The NIH-funded Center for Computational Mass Spectrometry at the University of California, San Diego, develops algorithms for large-scale analyses of mass spectrometry data and for two prominent service platforms for sharing mass spectrometry data. One platform is the Mass Spectrometry Interactive Virtual Environment,[11] which contains more than 10,000 data sets that are assigned identifiers and shared in conjunction with publications. The other platform is the Proteomics Scalable, Accessible, and Flexible environment[12] with more than 80 data analysis workflows. Bandeira noted that one of the Center's key tasks is to develop tools to analyze and increase the value of data,[13] which leads to the creation of new knowledge. Computer infrastructure and communities are needed to understand how data can be used to connect researchers who might unknowingly be working on related problems.

Bandeira noted that before discussing cost, it is imperative to develop domain-specific standards to determine what constitutes high-quality reusable data. A data set's storage value for future research can be determined by its uniqueness and its potential for additional discoveries. He added that it is important to develop platforms that will engage researchers in an ongoing curation process (i.e., the data that are available are automatically integrated into ongoing research projects, and reanalysis goes back into the curation of the data in the repository). This type of centralized platform is a departure from the traditional repository model

---

[11] For more information about the Mass Spectrometry Interactive Virtual Environment, see http://massive.ucsd.edu, accessed September 25, 2019.

[12] For more information about the Proteomics Scalable, Accessible, and Flexible environment, see http://proteomics.ucsd.edu/ProteoSAFe, accessed September 25, 2019.

[13] For more information about the software tools developed at the Center for Computational Mass Spectrometry, see http://proteomics.ucsd.edu/software, accessed September 25, 2019.

and promotes the exchange of knowledge as well as crowdsourcing to annotate data.

Tenenbaum stressed the value of user-friendly interfaces, visualization, and discoverability. Having worked on a large-scale community-based biorepository and registry of data (the Measurement to Understand the Reclassification of Disease of Cabarrus/Kannapolis study[14]), she noted that even experts are challenged with understanding relevant standards and what it means to annotate data. Her research group extracts symptom-related terms from electronic health record (EHR) data, which can be clustered for an analysis to understand underlying mechanisms of disease. She explained that curating, interacting with patients, obtaining consents, recruiting, and following-up are all important but expensive research activities. Thus, it is crucial to leverage data that are collected through clinical care and "build a learning health care system." Working with structured mental health data and text includes access to fully identified, highly sensitive clinical data. One error could inadvertently expose these data or cause problems in the data analysis and the resulting documentation.

Tenenbaum commented that tools for calculating potential costs for storage would be helpful for researchers. A clarification of rules and clear policies would also be beneficial—for example, experts currently disagree about what is considered to be a breach of the Health Insurance Portability and Accountability Act (HIPAA). She noted that grant budgets should include specific descriptions for tracking lifetime data costs. She also suggested an incentive system in which people who do not share data are either prevented from securing an indexed publication in PubMed or are added to a "wall of shame" ("sticks"), while people who exhibit best practices receive recognition ("carrots"). She cautioned that adding components to an already requirement-laden grant proposal process could create additional challenges.

Georgia (Gina) Tourassi, Oak Ridge National Laboratory, explained that the big data revolution in biomedical science began in radiology. She added that the U.S. Department of Energy (DOE) laboratories pride themselves on being stewards of data and tools across various domains. For example, in a partnership between DOE and the National Cancer Institute, Tourassi explores the use of high-performance computing and large-scale data analytics on cancer registry data—70 percent of data collected across cancer registries is text data that need to be curated. Artificial

---

[14] For more information about the Measurement to Understand the Reclassification of Disease of Cabarrus/Kannapolis study, see https://globalhealth.duke.edu/projects/measurement-understand-reclassification-disease-cabarruskannapolis-study-murdock, accessed October 8, 2019.

intelligence technologies can be used to abstract information from the data, and computational models of patient trajectories can be developed. The ultimate goal is to deliver tools to data owners (in this case, the cancer registries) and to distribute and scale algorithms that will enable them to train their own data using open compute resources. She emphasized that advances in biomedical science arise from using various data modalities to present a holistic view of a patient. However, it is challenging to do scalable data-driven discovery with heterogeneous data sources, including nontraditional data sets that could provide additional insights into patient care.

Tourassi wondered about the cost of data storage versus the cost of data analysis. Although colocating compute and data can make workflow and data management more feasible and more cost-effective, continued infrastructure investments are necessary. Questions also remain about the ownership of patient data and their derivatives as well as the legal responsibility for the deidentification of data. Hardware, software, and algorithmic approaches to enable collaboration are needed, as are increased incentives to share data. She reiterated Bandeira's assertion that the value of data will determine cost. Tourassi concluded by emphasizing the value of sustained infrastructure investment, which can advance innovation, support scientific discovery, and improve clinical practice.

Robert Williams, University of Tennessee Health Science Center, began his career with a study of brain architecture, which demanded a global approach and the integration of data with primitive tools such as Excel, FileMaker, and FileVision. After collecting data for 7 years, he received funding from the Human Brain Project to scale up his efforts. His primary objective is to enhance precision medicine by building animal model resources (in addition to human cohorts) that allow the incorporation of genetic diversity into mice and rats. He asserted that if data sit in a silo and cannot be correlated to anything, they are not of high value. However, if data can be acquired in a multiscalar way, as Ferguson described, additional vectors of data become multiplicative; in order for this to work computationally, web services and other tools have to be developed.

Williams said that open source code tools are useful, but they can be unpredictable. He emphasized that low-cost, secure enclaves are needed for protected health information, EHRs, and genomes to capture long-tail data. Encryption technologies that still allow data to be computable are also essential. He noted that both "carrots and sticks" should be used to motivate researchers to manage data and costs. However, he acknowledged that it is difficult to make predictions and develop solutions in a highly changeable environment. He asserted that while data loss and cost are problematic, capturing missing information (i.e., initial data, metadata) is a more immediate concern. He mentioned the importance of motivating researchers to use the InterPlanetary File System[15] and to have reputable workflows (e.g., via Guix, Galaxy, Jupyter, Open Science Foundation). Ultimately, he said, researchers should push against static publications (and move to Jupyter or R Shiny), allowing the data to "breathe and breed." The scientific culture needs to move away from primarily storytelling: Journal readers need to be able to read the narrative, see the data, and validate the narrative in real time.

Levenstein reiterated that the goal of the National Academies' study is to help researchers and funders better integrate risk management. She pointed out that all of the panelists mentioned an element of risk related to privacy and confidentiality, and she wondered about the following:

1. What do researchers need to be able to forecast risks and costs in grant proposals?
2. How can researchers think simultaneously about the cost of computing and the cost of preserving data?
3. What are the incentives for researchers to share data and manage risks? Which "carrots and sticks" resonate most with researchers?
4. Can economic and cultural standards change so that researchers willingly take on the costs of making their data available?

Bandeira described data as "having a life of their own" after an initial narrative is published. Therefore, to accurately assess curation costs, he said that it is important to think about data as a work in progress instead of as an end product. He added that if an investigator can use the same platform for both data analysis and data sharing, incentives increase and costs decrease. The Center for Computational Mass Spectrometry's systems offer continuous reanalysis of data; as new knowledge becomes available, it is automatically transferred to the data sets over the course of a project, thus reducing the data analysis burden for researchers and connecting them to other researchers with overlapping data sets. Levenstein championed the role of data sharing in community building, especially for interdisciplinary research.

Tourassi said that the cost of data storage is expected to continue to decrease but computing costs can vary by domain. Moving data can also require substantial investments in both time and money; thus, costs need to be evaluated early in the process, especially for projects that require continuous data movement. Capital, operational, and maintenance expenditures need to be considered when building and sustaining an infrastructure that can keep pace with evolving software and operating systems. To

---

[15] For more information about the InterPlanetary File System, see ipfs.io, accessed December 5, 2019.

avoid burdening researchers with software engineering, she suggested bringing scientists and engineers together to create a sustainable ecosystem. An online participant commented that technologists who maintain the operating systems of infrastructure are often the same people who maintain the technological capabilities for the rest of an organization. This participant wondered about the costs for such a model and whether it is sustainable for data maintenance. The participant added that without the right incentives, organizational-level information-technology teams could become barriers instead of enablers, prompting researchers to take things into their own hands.

Levenstein noted that data are active resources that extend beyond FAIR principles, thus creating both challenges and opportunities for the future. Tenenbaum asserted that financial risks and privacy risks are not mutually exclusive—when a breach occurs, both types of risk are realized—and noted that data provenance is another area in which to consider risk. Altintas emphasized the need for NLM to consider the risks and costs associated with data sharing and supported the development of a neutral cross-agency strategy to address health and privacy risks for the future of science. She asked panelists about their visions for the future. Tenenbaum suggested increased public–private partnerships; however, she recognized that this would add another layer of complexity to an already complicated process. Tourassi described the challenges of working with data across registries, including registry-specific restrictions as well as multiple memoranda of understanding, data use agreements, and business associate agreements. Additional complexities arise in private partnerships, particularly in terms of the ownership of intellectual property. A neutral entity could deploy centralized models to each registry to enable data sharing across registries (i.e., knowledge would be shared without each registry seeing the others' data). Bandeira pointed out that it is difficult to analyze heterogeneous data from different siloes, which in turn affects the data's value. He said that it is not necessary for one repository to have both the expertise to manage a particular data type and the ability to store and compute those data. There should be one place where all of the data can be stored, but the different entities that manage each data type and repository are still research endeavors that should be awarded separately. This approach dissociates the compute and storage capabilities from the infrastructure needed to organize, process, and connect data. An interoperable platform would bring the tools, data, and computing capabilities together, better connecting tool developers with the research. Because privacy will always be a concern, Tenenbaum suggested the increased use of application programming interfaces (APIs) to share *information* (as opposed to data). Tourassi noted that in her partnership with the National Cancer Surveillance program, tools are being built and deployed in the form of APIs. Such an ecosystem makes it possible to offer both open and restricted access. She added that it is important to consider the potential for adversarial use of algorithms; a benchmarking process could help determine the accuracy and vulnerability of algorithms to this misuse.

In response to a question from Martone, Bandeira said that any proteomics data that were assigned identifiers can be found in the ProteomeXchange consortium. With the emergence of tools that allow for joint analysis, there is an influx of transcriptomics data surfacing alongside the proteomics data. Martone wondered how repositories could communicate and coordinate in the absence of a centralized entity, and Bandeira noted that replication would be unavoidable.

Martone asked the panelists how career and grant cycles drive costs for and decisions about data. Tenenbaum said that the cycle itself provides the "carrot" for researchers to document metadata, which makes it possible for a project to continue even after a graduate student or other researcher departs. Williams added that his team typically prioritizes generating high-quality data over creating a narrative. Tourassi suggested employing a data manager and a software engineer for each project. Creating a culture of good practices requires support from the top down, she continued. Bandeira said that for long-term projects, data sets should be available for follow-up analysis and independent reanalysis. With the right tools to enable data sharing, he said that data will improve with age and become enduring resources for the research community.

3

Data Risks and Costs

**PANEL DISCUSSION: ADDRESSING DATA
RISKS AND THEIR COSTS**

*Michelle Meyer, Geisinger, Moderator
Amy O'Hara, Georgetown University
Brad Malin, Vanderbilt University Medical Center
Trevor Owens, U.S. Library of Congress*

Serving as moderator for this panel discussion, Michelle Meyer, Geisinger, explained that the management of data risks and their costs requires a discussion of data integrity, data usability and operability, privacy and security, and accessibility as well as consideration for the challenges around establishing and enforcing appropriate terms of data use. Amy O'Hara, Georgetown University, discussed strategies to manage the risks associated with acquiring, managing, and curating data. She explained that because data use can result in financial, legal, social, and emotional costs, it is imperative to create data use agreements. There are risks associated with establishing data use agreements, keeping them in place, and enforcing them as data are used over time. The first step is to build trust between data producers and data users. Data use agreements codify terms and conditions (e.g., how the data will be moved and whether signatories are needed for modifications) to ensure that each party interacts with the data responsibly. This trusted relationship is jeopardized if data producers withdraw from the agreement or if data users fail to deliver the intended value of the data. In order to enforce a data agreement, she continued, the terms of use have to be clear, especially regarding subsequent data use, and an authority has to be defined who will approve and explain the agreement and foster continued responsible use of data. To best manage these risks when establishing and maintaining data use agreements, it is crucial to develop templates, understand where legal precedent exists, and clearly communicate in language that all parties understand. She described the data agreement itself as metadata that should be linked to the data sets and to the publication—this supports the scientific integrity of a study as well as future responsible research.

O'Hara cautioned that it is important to understand the difference between a legally binding contract and an agreement—for example, contracts for the purchase of commercial data could have more complicated terms of use than data agreements with federal or state entities. Additional questions related to liability can arise: How are data being managed? Who is liable if the data are used beyond the scope of the terms of the agreement? Whoever has access to personal identifiers will need to be able to handle them responsibly and uniformly. O'Hara championed the vision of implementing a federated data system with trained, documented, and trusted brokers to facilitate the linkage of data. However, she emphasized the need to consider how records will be purged, as well as how synthetic data will be managed, before developing and implementing such a system.

O'Hara hopes that data intermediaries will help data producers understand their responsibility to produce metadata and to enforce responsible, secure uses of data. Smart contracts, in which the terms of use are encoded, could be useful for data management in the future. A thorough understanding of legal precedents is required for this approach; however, with more automation, it could be possible to reduce the number of humans in the loop and the amount of human error.

Brad Malin, Vanderbilt University Medical Center, described the explicit and implicit costs of privacy. He noted that in the mid-1990s, it became apparent that diagnostics, costs, procedures, and individuals' demographic data were needed to do comparative effectiveness research to improve health care. However, these types of data are linkable to other resources that contain individuals' identities (see Figure 3.1).

He recounted the experience of William Weld, governor of Massachusetts from 1991 to 1997, to illuminate the problem with quasi-identifiers. After Weld was admitted to Massachusetts General Hospital, it was possible to identify him with only the knowledge of his full 5-digit zip code, gender, full date of birth, and approximate time of admittance. This instance led to the discussion of deidentification in the Health Insurance Portability and Accountability Act (HIPAA), which clarifies that full 5-digit zip codes and full dates of birth are potentially identifiable. Weld's

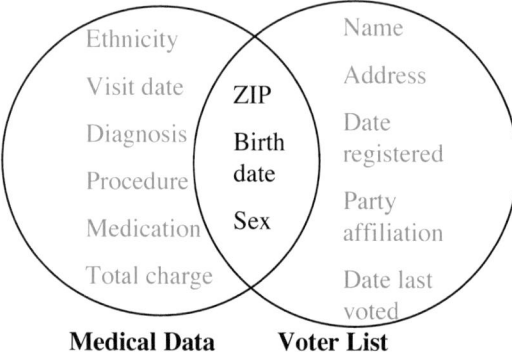

FIGURE 3.1 The quasi-identifier conundrum. SOURCE: Republished with permission of *International Journal on Uncertainty, Fuzziness and Knowledge-based Systems*, from L. Sweeney, k-anonymity: A model for protecting privacy, *International Journal on Uncertainty, Fuzziness and Knowledge-based Systems* 10:5, 2002; permission conveyed through Copyright Clearance Center, Inc.

case was not an exception: with knowledge of zip codes, birth dates, and genders, the majority of people in the United States can be uniquely identified.

Malin referenced America Online as a cautionary tale of the cost implications of privacy violations. America Online monitored people's movements online, viewed their queries, captured the links they were clicking, and made clickstream data publicly accessible—sharing data on the search queries of 650,000 customers. The only precaution taken was to replace the names of the individuals with persistent pseudonyms (in the form of user numbers). With the help of computer scientists, two investigative journalists at the *New York Times* were able to use these data to identify user number 4417749, and a $10 million class-action lawsuit was filed shortly thereafter. However, similar cases continued to surface. In 2009, a class-action lawsuit was filed against Netflix after it shared data on the movie selections of 450,000 individuals—despite the use of pseudonyms, reidentification was still possible. As a result, the company has not shared any user data in the past 10 years. He emphasized that although reidentification is possible with nearly any feature, it will not happen in practice on every occasion.

The National Institutes of Health's All of Us Research Program has adopted a tiered-access approach to data sharing, Malin explained. This approach includes a public access model, in which aggregate statistics about individuals are shared. It also includes two tiers of sandbox environments on Google Cloud: In the registered tier, select people will be given access to individual-level records with minimal risk of participant identification. The controlled tier contains the individual-level records with greater risk of participant identification; however, the overall risk is expected to be low because the number of people with access to the controlled tier (all of whom are carefully vetted) is significantly reduced.

Malin stated that individuals are driven by incentives both to share and to exploit data. The cost to access data and the level at which they can be accessed vary by state; in Weld's case, data were inexpensive and easy to exploit. Malin's team modeled this scenario as a strategic 2-party privacy game between the publisher and the recipient; essentially, various data-sharing strategies (e.g., generalizing demographics, perturbing statistics, applying data use agreements, charging for access) are attacked to expose the risks. This privacy game reveals which data-sharing strategy optimizes the risk-utility trade-off to aid in decision making. He emphasized that deidentification is not a panacea; the risk of reidentification exists in any security setting. Thus, the best path forward is to determine an appropriate level of risk and to ensure accountability in a system. He agreed with O'Hara that one should never share data without a data use agreement in place and that risk is proportional to the anticipated trustworthiness of the recipient. He noted that because there are many ways to manipulate data, people have proposed alternate data protection frameworks such as encrypted computation, secure hardware, and blockchain. However, blockchain was not designed to protect privacy; it only provides the lineage of those who worked with the data. He also expressed concern about moving to a particular encryption system or to a centralized server, which could lead to technology lock-in. He explained that deidentification results in a loss of data utility; encryption results in a loss of functionality; and secure environments result in a loss in efficiency. However, with no action, the potential outcomes include losses of privacy, money (due to litigation and remuneration), societal trust, and scientific opportunity.

Trevor Owens, U.S. Library of Congress, described the foundational risks associated with digital preservation. Identifying and responding to risks related to loss of access and use is the first step to ensuring long-term access to digital content. He explained that the National Digital Stewardship Alliance (NDSA)[1] has established the Levels of Digital Preservation, which provide recommendations to approach planning and policy development for digital preservation (see Phillips et al., 2013). He described the Levels of Digital Preservation as similar to the Trustworthy Repositories

---

[1] For more information about NDSA, see ndsa.org, accessed October 1, 2019.

Audit and Certification: Criteria and Checklist (TRAC),[2] although the TRAC standard focuses more on the policy frameworks that are required to enable the development of a digital preservation infrastructure. The NDSA Levels have tiered guidance, anchored in the notion that digital preservation is never complete.

Owens described the five risk areas outlined in the Levels of Digital Preservation:

1. *Storage and geographic location of the data.* To mitigate the risk that damage to storage media could result in a total loss of data, multiple copies of the data should be managed in various geographic regions with different disaster threats.
2. *File fixity and data integrity.* To avoid losing data through use, transactions, or bit rot (i.e., data at rest can degrade on storage media), fixity information should be generated, tracked, logged, and managed across copies (e.g., through cryptographic caches). It is also important to repair bad copies of data.
3. *Information security.* To avoid losing data through unauthorized user actions, access restrictions should be managed, actions on files should be logged, and logs should be audited to ensure that the actions taken were intended.
4. *Metadata.* To prevent the loss of the usability of data or the ability to authenticate data, administrative, technical, descriptive, and preservation metadata should be produced and managed, and non-colocated copies of metadata should be maintained.
5. *File formats.* To avoid the loss of usability or renderability of data, the following actions should be taken: articulate preservation intention, limit format support in terms of sustainability factors, take inventory of formats, validate files, produce derivatives, and use virtualization and emulation technologies to enable data use. File formats present the biggest challenge for long-term planning.

Owens suggested that the best way to mitigate these risks is to have permanent trained staff working in these areas and to plan a continual refresh cycle of software and hardware. He added that these initiatives should not be supported by project-based funding but rather as a central cost. Each time that researchers work with digital materials, a new set of costs arises to ensure continuity and accessibility of those materials. To gauge an organization's level of commitment to digital preservation, Owens suggested asking the organization's accountants the following

---

[2] For more information about TRAC, see https://www.crl.edu/archiving-preservation/digital-archives/metrics-assessing-and-certifying/trac, accessed October 1, 2019.

question: What part of core operations resources are invested in staffing, contracts, software, and hardware dedicated to digital preservation?

Owens said that the Levels of Digital Preservation have been widely adopted, and academic institutions have found them particularly useful in performing a quick check to understand which risks are of immediate concern and which could better drive long-term investments. David Maier, Portland State University, pointed out that the Levels of Digital Preservation do not account for the fundamental risk that preservation could fail simply owing to a lack of resources. Owens replied that because costs on base-level bit-preservation work are relatively low, an imminent threat of losing the data can be avoided. In cases in which there are not enough resources to meet the bare minimum, Owens suggested asking the organization if it is committed to preservation and discussing what types of resources are needed to ensure long-term access. Historically, the data that have actually been collected and managed have only been a fraction of what could have been kept or managed. Categorizing data into the right areas in terms of the consequences of loss has to become part of cost modeling, he asserted.

Ilkay Altintas, University of California, San Diego, said that data science education programs rely on the opportunity to train students with real data sets and/or anonymized industry data sets to best prepare them to enter the workforce. She wondered how to balance this educational need with privacy concerns. Malin said that the question of who should have access to data and how that access should be given is complicated. He added that processes (e.g., rounding out outliers) to ensure that an individual cannot be identified reduce the fidelity of data, which might prove unhelpful for certain research questions. O'Hara said that a data use agreement could specify that all data users sign a nondisclosure agreement. Privacy protections for disseminated data could also be built directly into such an agreement. Malin noted that data agreements only extend so far because even if a person does not *disclose* the reidentification, it still occurs. He added that once data are labeled as "deidentified," the federal government cannot step in and enforce a regulation. In that case, people rely on civil contractual agreements.

Lars Vilhuber, Cornell University, asked about mechanisms to create incentivized data provision agreements. O'Hara said that both publishers and funders have operable levers to incentivize researchers to share data. She agreed with Malin that much of the role of making incentives more visible and equitable, however, falls to government entities. Vilhuber wondered if there is an intermediate incentive to increase data sharing between the motivation to be a good citizen and the threat of a federal regulation. O'Hara said that data united at the state level for an operational need or for compliance reporting builds trust and incentivizes the use of data more broadly. Malin added that coregulatory models exist outside of the United States; in those cases, the rules for data sharing are enforced by a consortium (e.g., industry and/or academia) instead of by the government.

SUMMARIES OF SMALL-GROUP DISCUSSIONS

Mechanisms for Forecasting the Costs of Maintained Privacy

Vilhuber explained that his group discussed ways to expand researchers' knowledge of privacy protection. The group also debated whether the university or the research community should support mechanisms to implement privacy models (e.g., tiered models, improved consent templates) and to better apply privacy-preserving techniques to data. He said that the group explored how universities currently address privacy-related issues. For example, do Institutional Review Boards have the necessary skills and tools to support researchers in the proper sharing of data and to evaluate the privacy design of a study? Considerations for the proper sharing of data should begin at the planning stage of a study, he noted. The group also discussed how to channel some of the market value of data back to study participants and how that relates to the notion of privacy. He added that privacy protocols should be communicated to participants.

Vilhuber pointed out that the university could alleviate some of the burdens on researchers, although concerns remain about unfunded mandates to scale such an approach. He mentioned a brief conversation among the group members about the value of dissemination plans; while they can add to the burden for researchers on the front end, they could ultimately lead to positive outcomes. The final topic considered by the group was the construction of a system (e.g., a new infrastructure for collaboration or discovery) that would give researchers an advantage. Protocol standardization is one way to reduce the friction of contributing to such platforms, Vilhuber explained.

Mechanisms for Identifying Risk and Cost Factors of Research Data in the Cloud

Maier explained that his group discussed data egress in relation to risks and costs of the cloud. Once data have been collected and stored, there is still continued cost when people access them. One way to address that issue is to adopt a requestor-pays model. However, that approach is not without risks: If a user has a limited amount of money to spend, he or she might run out of funds before a particular computation finishes. Maier noted that some states and municipal governments already have preferred cloud providers, which means that it is difficult for an individual within one of those government agencies to receive permission or funding to use data in a different cloud. He explained that the group was unaware of any current cloud-agnostic solution that would allow an individual to select whatever provider his or her agency approved. If there is a need to change providers, large costs result both for data egress and data ingress. To address that problem, he continued, in-house copies of the data can be maintained (i.e., it is often easier to re-provision on a new platform from an in-house copy than to move between platforms).

Maier raised a question that emerged during the group discussion: If certain security mechanisms and restrictions have been implemented on the data themselves, and one goes to the cloud to compute with them, would the compute platform observe the same security protocols as those used for storage? He noted that data sets that are covered by different licenses are becoming more freely available and combined more often. The group also discussed certain regulatory regimes, privacy laws, and consumer protection laws that could prohibit the placement of data in certain geographic locations. He added that if the security requirements for federal use of the cloud (i.e., the Federal Risk and Authorization Management Program) change substantially, there might be additional burden for providers and an increase of cost to use that service. An influx of questions and requests for help could also result from successful use of a data set (even one for which people pay), a burden which could deter investigators from placing their data on a particular platform.

Mechanisms for Identifying the Costs of Making Data Truly Findable

Margaret Levenstein, University of Michigan, summarized her group's conversation about what it would cost to make data more findable in the future. She said that tools are needed to make it easier for researchers to curate data during the research process. She also suggested that the grant process should change, perhaps with the addition of a new section that would require researchers to disclose any prior data that they had collected, not just prior research that they had conducted. Levenstein described this proposal as "actionable and impactful" because it justifies the need for new data collection. The group also discussed ways to enforce funders' requirements for data sharing. She suggested that there would be value in implementing training at the beginning of a grant; then, at the end of a grant, principal investigators would be able to compare actual costs to costs forecasted in their data management plans.

Levenstein also suggested the need to link data and publications more consistently. She noted the group's conversation about creating a PubMed that would link to repositories where the data reside as well as developing a centralized registry of repositories and metadata sources. Training is needed for newly created repositories to ensure that they foster best practices, use existing standards, and build communities. She emphasized the need to train people across disciplines to build on and sustain work that has already been done. In response to a question from Patricia Flatley Brennan, National Library of Medicine, Levenstein said that although there was much group discussion about how to meet standards, there was no discussion about common data elements.

4

Tools and Practices for Risk Management, Data Preservation, and Accessing Decisions

DATA—WHAT'S IT GOING TO COST, AND WHAT'S IN IT FOR ME?

Philip Bourne, University of Virginia

Philip Bourne, University of Virginia, described an ongoing fundamental shift in academia, particularly around the notion of data science. However, he noted that data science has been part of biomedicine for several years, starting with the creation of the Human Genome Project. He expects that other disciplines (e.g., religious studies, politics, and environmental science) will also embrace data science and explained that members of the biomedical community can both teach these disciplines and learn from them moving forward.

He discussed the various stakeholders in data supply chains: Funders contribute to the development of resources, publishers provide resources to both readers and authors, the National Institutes of Health (NIH) impacts researchers, and university deans and presidents guide faculty and students. He emphasized that neither the institution of higher education itself nor these supply chains are sustainable in their current forms. Bourne described the Protein Data Bank (PDB), a research collaboratory for structured bioinformatics, as "an exemplar of biological resources." PDB is run on a 5-year funding cycle with no guarantee that it will be funded for the next 5-year increment, despite the fact that the PDB has more than 1 million users each year and it would cost $14 billion to recreate its contents. He said that there was a reluctance on the part of developers of the PDB to seek private funding for fear that doing so would reduce federal funding and destabilize the project. This raises questions about the value of resources that exist under a tenuous model. This level of uncertainty also prompts people to leave academia for careers in industry, where incentives and stability are more prominent. Thus, people and resources that are fundamental to underlying science should be sustained appropriately, he asserted. He added that increased international cooperation is needed at the funding level of the supply chain.

Bourne turned to a discussion of publishers' involvement in the data supply chain. He noted that data are being maintained by publishers, but only large publishers can sustain a data ecosystem. For example, the Public Library of Science (PLOS) requires authors to deposit their data in a repository in order to publish. However, PLOS does not have the expertise or resources to maintain a repository, so it proposed the use of FigShare and Dryad. It remains to be seen whether these approaches are reliable and sustainable, Bourne explained. He also pointed out that PubMed is now including and supporting data because data sets that are aggregated are more useful than a single data set.

In the NIH and university portions of the data supply chain, Bourne observed that the difference between data science and data management needs to be clarified. He also suggested that the distinction between computational and experimental research be eliminated, as the next generation of researchers will have crosscutting skill sets. Alternative business models and an increased emphasis on data management plans would also be beneficial. For example, researchers should begin to acknowledge their funding source(s) when posting data in a repository (which could then be searched as metadata), thus revealing whether they have complied with their data management plans. He asserted that university administrators might not fully appreciate the value of data and how important data access is to the future success of their institutions. Faculty and students, in turn, often lack appropriate access even to their own data.

Bourne explained that there is a new level of disruption as a result of digitization. He described future drivers of change, including the fact that there are more data available than people know what to do with and the demand continues to grow. Tools have improved dramatically (e.g., Python, R, deep artificial neural networks) and have become more robust and reusable, computing power has increased, and training data are doubling every 2 years. Many of these improvements are happening in the private sector but not in academia, he noted.

Bourne predicted that it is going to become even more difficult to forecast data costs in the coming years. Sharing an anecdote about a trauma surgeon who sought correlations between public vehicle crash data and electronic health records data that would allow him to better treat future patients, Bourne emphasized data integration of diverse data by new types of researchers can lead to important biomedical outcomes. He noted the need to preserve data collectively to enhance reproducibility; however, in the case of the trauma surgeon, no suitable repository exists to sustain his work.

Unique opportunities are emerging in higher education—for example, the University of Virginia is establishing a new school of data science, and nearly 200 U.S. postsecondary institutions offer some form of data science training. Although postsecondary institutions are training excellent data scientists, they have no way to retain them as employees. He asserted that the institutional culture around data needs to change. Postsecondary institutions need to use their own data effectively to improve productivity. He emphasized the importance of rewarding reproducible science and open science in which data play a prominent role—via the faculty/staff handbook, the hiring process, and the promotion process. He explained that the university library also plays a critical role, working across the institution and moving from data preservationist to data analyst. He noted the need for better data governance in postsecondary institutions to manage metadata and data sharing—it is imperative that postsecondary institutions develop an infrastructure for moving data, moving from siloes to commons-like environments. Postsecondary institutions can thus relieve the burden from federal funders and begin to maintain more useful research output through a combination of (1) internal resources (i.e., if reference data sets and quality data can be used year after year by incoming students, they could be supported by tuition funds), (2) federal funding, (3) philanthropy, and (4) public–private partnerships (e.g., relationships can begin via student capstone experiences, which generate data, larger projects, and a talent pipeline).

Bourne highlighted the "data deluge and opportunities lost" in cost forecasting. Bourne said that data preservation can cost as much as people are willing to spend. He said that because the demand (science) far outweighs the supply (data resources), it is important to support the resources that make the most strategic sense (e.g., foster public–private relationships and give postsecondary institutions and the private sector more responsibility for data). If data are considered part of a broader ecosystem with many stakeholders, costs will decrease, research will improve, and health care will advance, he asserted. He posed the following questions for participants to consider throughout the rest of the workshop: What role do you think postsecondary institutions and the private sector should play in the support of data? Does the emergence of data science present opportunities?

David Chu, Institute for Defense Analyses, asked Bourne how he has dealt with the private sector's desire to retain ownership of its data.

Bourne said that in some partnerships, students have to sign contracts to transfer the intellectual property. That approach, however, encourages the use of synthetic data. Maryann Martone, University of California, San Diego, observed that data ownership policies in many postsecondary institutions have not been revised in more than 50 years, which creates confusion among researchers about data responsibility, ownership, and stewardship. Bourne agreed with the urgent need to update university data policies and commended those institutions that have hired chief data officers. Resources such as the PDB are assets that attract strong faculty candidates—in the future, the value of a postsecondary institution will be directly related to the data assets it has and makes public, he commented. Sarah Nusser, Iowa State University, said that transformations are needed in academia and for research practice more broadly. She wondered what role a postsecondary institution and, more specifically, the library would play in helping researchers prepare to share data. Bourne said that faculty researchers will think more about the value of data and the need to provide metadata when they are evaluated by how much data they share and their degree of cooperation. When students begin to use those data and credit the use to those researchers, a new wave of data sharing could begin within a postsecondary institution.

Nuno Bandeira, University of California, San Diego, explained that as postsecondary institutions begin to embrace data, metrics will be needed to assess the value of data sets and database interaction. Bourne said that if good data citation practices are in place, standard bibliometric techniques could be used to determine the number of citations given to data sets. People should have the opportunity to evaluate data in the same way that they can evaluate narratives, he added. Monica McCormick, University of Delaware Library, cautioned about making intellectual property agreements with publishers that are becoming data analytics firms. Bourne wholeheartedly agreed, emphasizing how discouraging it would be if researchers had to buy back their own data because they had not managed them properly.

PRECISELY PRACTICING MEDICINE FROM 700 TRILLION POINTS OF DATA

Atul Butte, University of California, San Francisco
(participating remotely)

Atul Butte, University of California, San Francisco, opened his presentation with a description of the National Center for Biotechnology Information (NCBI) Gene Expression Omnibus and the European Bioinformatics

Institute (EBI) ArrayExpress.[1] In 2012, these two data archives collectively contained 1 million samples; they now already contain more than 2.25 million samples. He noted that NCBI provides access to this information without even requiring users to use a username or password. He remarked on the successes of several open data repositories. For example, The Cancer Genome Atlas[2] references more than 14,000 cases across 39 types of cancers and includes 13 types of data (e.g., molecular, clinical, and sequencing), some of which are accessible at various levels. Genetics researchers also share a vast array of data via the Database of Genotypes and Phenotypes (dbGaP),[3] access to which requires the completion of paperwork and an occasional Institutional Review Board application. Chemical biologists use PubChem[4] to share their data, which references 227 million substances, 1.3 million assays, and more than 1 billion measurements within a grid of 300 trillion cells. Molecular biologists share their data via ENCODE,[5] which has 442 principal investigators across 32 institutes and 15 TB of data.

Butte explained that immunologists and clinical trialists also share their data. For example, with nearly 400 data sets and approximately 1,000 users each month, ImmPort[6] is likely the largest repository for flow cytometry data and the one repository that allows raw, deidentified clinical trials data to be downloaded by the public. ImmPort has expanded by collecting data beyond the National Institutes of Health—for example, vaccine data from the Bill and Melinda Gates Foundation and preterm birth data from the March of Dimes. He noted that all requests for applications (RFAs) from the National Institute of Allergy and Infectious Diseases (NIAID) require researchers to deposit data to ImmPort. NIAID also offers funding to download and use data from ImmPort. He proposed that NIH continue to develop RFAs with similar requirements in the future. Google Cloud, which contains many high-level data sets (e.g., population health, Centers for Disease Control data, Centers for Medicaid and Medicare Services data, Google Data Set Search), provides another avenue for data sharing. He wondered why so few researchers take advantage of all of

---

[1] For more information about ArrayExpress, see https://www.ebi.ac.uk/arrayexpress, accessed September 25, 2019.

[2] For more information about The Cancer Genome Atlas, see https://www.cancer.gov/about-nci/organization/ccg/research/structural-genomics/tcga, accessed October 1, 2019.

[3] For more information about the Database of Genotypes and Phenotypes, see https://www.ncbi.nlm.nih.gov/gap, accessed October 1, 2019.

[4] For more information about PubChem, see https://pubchem.ncbi.nlm.nih.gov, accessed October 1, 2019.

[5] For more information about ENCODE, see https://www.encodeproject.org, accessed October 1, 2019.

[6] For more information about ImmPort, see https://www.immport.org/home, accessed October 1, 2019.

these available data for experiments that could identify new drugs for patients.

Butte suggested that postsecondary institutions become more involved in motivating researchers to share data. For example, with assistance from the campus library, the University of California, San Francisco, distributes citable Digital Object Identifiers so that researchers can make their data publicly available. The entire University of California system utilizes a digital library system, which provides open access guidelines for publication. He asserted that researchers will not be convinced to change their behavior and share data with the motivation of citation or promotion alone.

Butte provided 10 reasons to archive and share study data openly:

1. Enhance reproducibility,
2. Improve transparency,
3. Support public policy,
4. Return data to the community,
5. Make failed trials and studies visible,
6. Enable learning,
7. Speed results reporting,
8. Enable new ventures,
9. Increase trust and believability, and
10. Develop new science.

He described the need to develop new science as the key driver for scientific data sharing. For example, ImmPort's 10,000 Immunome Project, which contains data on 10,000 people in control groups from clinical trials, generates a multiethnic, multirace, multiage, and multigender representation of a normal healthy immune system (see Figure 4.1).

Butte shared three anecdotes about the value of shared data. He noted that because preeclampsia screening was inadequate, his team sought to develop a more precise diagnostic tool for the potentially lethal condition. The team searched NCBI's Gene Expression Omnibus and EBI's ArrayExpress, found dozens of experiments with hundreds of samples, looked for commonalities and repeating patterns, and conducted tests. The result of this research was the spin-out and formation of Carmenta Bioscience after $2 million in seed funding was raised. A second study was inspired by the high costs (e.g., between $4 billion and $12 billion) associated with developing new drugs. The PubChem and the NIH Library of Integrated Network-Based Cellular Signatures[7] repositories have data that can be

---

[7] For more information on the Library of Integrated Network-Based Cellular Signatures, see http://www.lincsproject.org, accessed October 1, 2019.

used to develop new drugs, find new uses for old drugs, and reposition drugs. Through computation and testing, his team identified a drug that could potentially be used to treat liver cancer. This work led to the development of another company, NuMedii, which has raised more than $10 million, continuing the research on drugs to treat other diseases. Lastly, with an interest in using genome sequencing to predict disease based on genetic polymorphisms, he co-founded the company Personalis—an endeavor that began with a high school student reading articles and has now successfully completed an Initial Purchase Offering, raising more than $200 million with approximately 150 employees.

Butte shared four important guidelines for building big data ecosystems: (1) sufficient data that can impact health care already exist (i.e., diagnostics and drugs can be developed from public big data), (2) extremely high-quality public and open data are readily available, (3) "sticks" seem to work better than "carrots" to motivate data sharing, and (4) the field needs more inquisitive researchers and trained students to initiate data science.

Chu asked Butte to elaborate on his perspective about strategies to motivate researchers to share data. Butte described a fundamental problem: Because the person who submits data often does not benefit in the same way as the person who uses data, it might be necessary to "force" or otherwise incentivize people to share their data. In addition, NIH program directors cannot be the ones responsible for enforcing data sharing because they have to maintain positive relationships with the best scientists from the best laboratories, he continued. Thus, another entity is needed to enforce data sharing. In that case, NIH can then work in partnership with the researchers to make the process as painless as possible. Patricia Flatley Brennan, National Library of Medicine, asked Butte whether charging people to reuse data would accelerate or decelerate research. Butte replied that researchers already pay for high-value data sets, but it is not a model that they appreciate. Alexa McCray, Harvard Medical School, pointed out that if there is a fee for the use of "high-value" data sets, free data will no longer be available and it will be impossible to aggregate across multiple data sets. Such a cost model could lead to discrimination against those who cannot pay as well as heterogeneity in the type of data that is available. Brennan asserted that grants provide a pathway to payment; direct pay is not a strategy that NIH has discussed. Martone pointed out that when a researcher pays for data, he or she has the right to redistribute them. Margaret Levenstein, University of Michigan, cautioned against creating processes that could make data access even more difficult for junior researchers. Bandeira reiterated that extraordinary value can be derived from data that already exist and asked how much of that value is returned to the community and shared publicly. Butte replied that none of the value is returned if no sharing mechanism (beyond articles) exists.

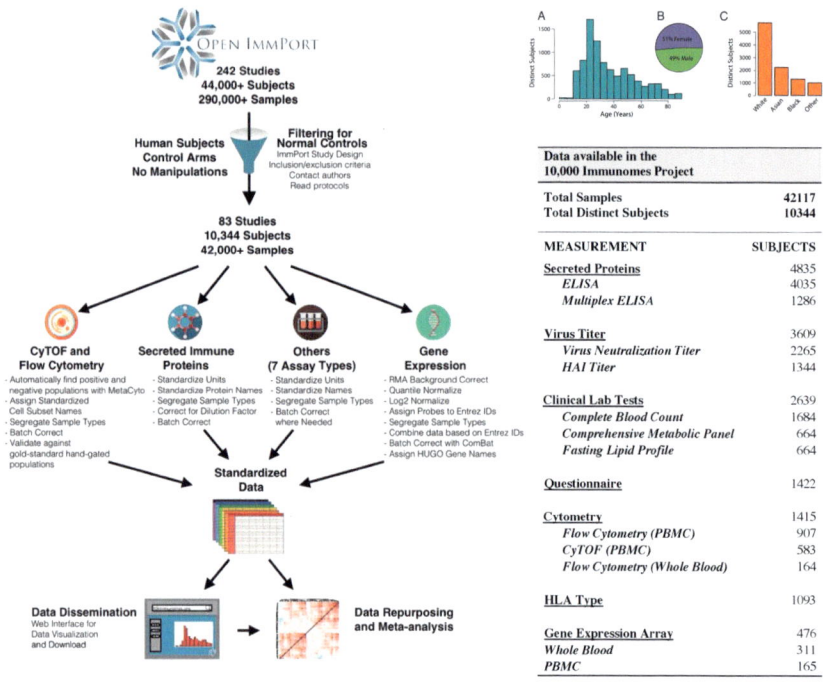

FIGURE 4.1 (*continues on following page*) The impacts of the Immunome project. SOURCE: Atul Butte, University of California, San Francisco, presentation to the workshop, July 11, 2019. Images available courtesy of CC-BY attribution license for K. Zalocusky, M.J. Kan, Z. Hu, P. Dunn, E. Thomson, J. Wiser, S. Bhattacharya, and A.J. Butte, The 10,000 Immunomes Project: Building a resource for human immunology, *Cell Reports* 25(2):513-522, 2018.

TOOLS AND PRACTICES FOR RISK MANAGEMENT

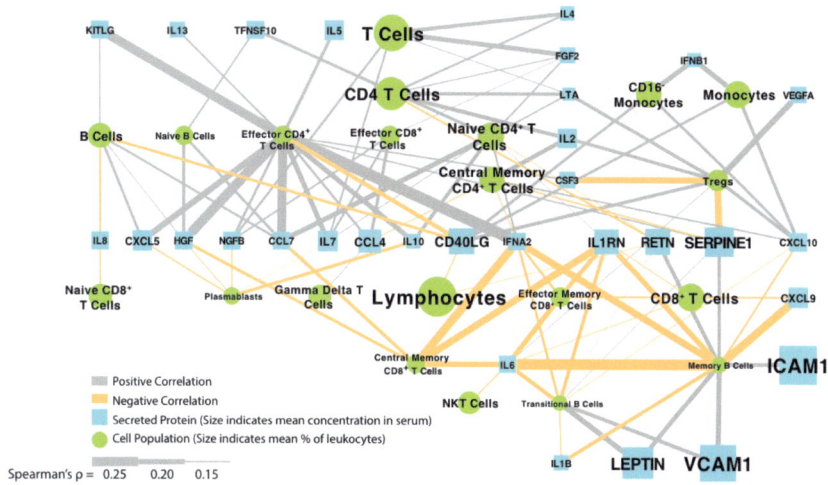

FIGURE 4.1 continued.

5

Lifetime Data Costs

To open the second day of the workshop, Alexa McCray, Harvard Medical School, summarized important messages from the first day of the workshop. She said that although data are not created equal, they improve when integrated with other data. Thus, it is essential that the most useful data are preserved. As a resource builds and obtains more data, scientists reclaim value, she continued. Questions remain about how to fund data sharing and preservation—if researchers can demonstrate that science advances as a direct result of sharing data via particular methods and platforms, an increase in long-term funding from the federal government and foundations could be justified.

PANEL DISCUSSION: INCENTIVES, MECHANISMS, AND PRACTICES FOR IMPROVED AWARENESS OF COST CONSEQUENCES IN DATA DECISIONS

Lars Vilhuber, Cornell University, Moderator
John Chodacki, University of California Curation Center, California Digital Library
Melissa Cragin, San Diego Supercomputer Center
Wendy Nilsen, National Science Foundation
Lucy Ofiesh, Center for Open Science

Panel moderator Lars Vilhuber, Cornell University, noted that in July 2019, the American Economic Association updated its data and code availability policy: Data will now be treated as primary objects, and authors will be required to submit to prepublication verification. However, publication is at the tail end of a research project, and researchers should think about the entire life cycle of research, starting from the conception of an idea to the final publication, he said, as well as the data reuse that might occur afterward.

John Chodacki, University of California Curation Center (UC3), California Digital Library (CDL), explained that UC3 focuses specifically on research data management, digital preservation, and persistent identifiers—part of a larger suite of services that CDL offers across the University of California system. Three years ago, CDL began to consider how to sustain the cost of preservation, what happens after successfully capturing research outputs, and ways in which campuses can get more involved. Although the campus community thinks carefully about how to set up computational environments and support computational research, his team recognized that the preservation policies, as well as plans to make data accessible and reusable over time, were merely ad hoc processes.

He described a pilot at CDL, with the entire University of California system, to address some of these data preservation issues. The pilot included stakeholders from across the campus communities, including the libraries, research entities, and information technology systems. Their goal was to make data more discoverable and more usable, while adhering to FAIR (findable, accessible, interoperable, reusable) principles, reducing hurdles for reuse and for advancement, and building capacity for researchers. The team agreed that storage costs needed to be addressed in this pilot—make upfront capital investments in storage, leverage storage across the system, and create a distributed storage network that is paid for through different budgets.

Chodacki said that while the pilot was ultimately unsuccessful, the process illuminated important lessons. Conversations with diverse stakeholders were crucial to convince three campuses to invest in purchasing or acquiring additional storage as well as to evaluate policies and procedures. One flaw in the pilot was its lack of researcher involvement; without an understanding of front-end processes, a pilot to improve back-end processes could not gain traction. Researchers need to be champions for these types of issues, but it was difficult to demonstrate the value of long-term preservation to researchers, he continued. The team also realized that pilots traditionally try to solve complex problems on a small scale; the pilot might have gained more traction had it been done on a larger scale. With further conversation about alternative approaches, UC3 connected with Dryad—a curated data repository that works across many fields and domains and accepts more than 300 GB per Digital Object Identifier—to discuss its potential support of institutional needs. A partnership with

Dryad emerged, and Dryad will now be offered to all University of California researchers at no cost.

CDL also works on issues related to machine-actionable data management plans (DMPs), which can be used to help model data preservation costs and understand those costs throughout the entire research life cycle. DMPTool,[1] a platform with 43 templates for 17 U.S. funders as well as international funders, is used by more than 31,000 researchers at 237 universities across the world. The tool is publicly available, and more than 250 campuses have a custom DMPTool. Chodacki's team has a grant from the National Science Foundation (NSF) to retrofit DMPTool and other DMP ecosystems to be more machine actionable. He explained that DMPs are active documents. To help with forecasting costs, DMPs need to expose structural information (including data volume) as a project progresses, make information available to the right parties, and be updateable by multiple parties in a decentralized fashion. Chodacki's team is working with DataCite's Event Data with Crossref as a means to use scholarly infrastructure to capture controlled information within a DMP and share it through an existing central hub. He emphasized that none of this work would be possible without collaboration: The team has been leveraging the Research Data Alliance[2] to build common standards for the format underlying machine-actionable DMPs (see Figure 5.1).

Melissa Cragin, San Diego Supercomputer Center, discussed ways to facilitate access to and use of active data (i.e., data within the research life cycle). She commended the "action leaders" in the United States and Europe (e.g., libraries, research computing departments, campus information technology specialists, and other administrators) who are seeking structural and process changes to encourage the management and stewardship of data within constrained budgets. Other constraints related to research data management include the breadth of services available, the relationships between technology and infrastructure platforms, and the transparency of ownership and costs. She explained that many faculty are interested in making their data available, learning about costs and trade-offs, and planning accordingly. Sustainable models are needed, she continued, which also requires commitment from campus leaders.

Cragin contacted colleagues from campuses across the United States and asked the following questions:

- What is happening on campus in terms of interactions with faculty to help them understand costing?

---

[1] For more information about the DMPTool, see Dmptool.org, accessed September 25, 2019.
[2] For more information about the Research Data Alliance, see rd-alliance.org, accessed September 25, 2019.

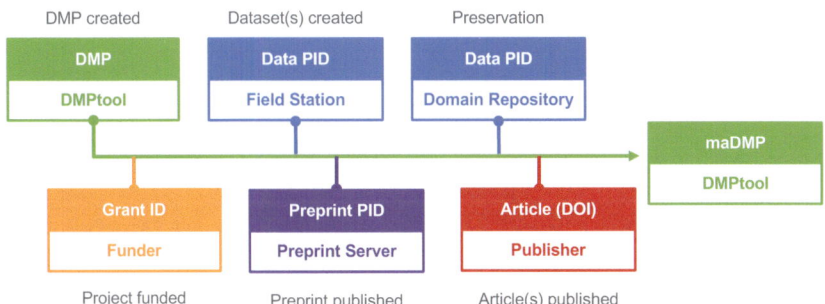

FIGURE 5.1 The path toward a machine-actionable data management plan. SOURCE: John Chodacki, University of California Curation Center, California Digital Library, presentation to the workshop, July 12, 2019.

- What processes are being used, and are there tools available?
- How are units collaborating, and is there infrastructure on campus?
- What are the costs? Where are they showing up? She described several examples into different service categories (see Table 5.1).

In the *unfunded linked-facilitator model*, the campus information technology center and the high-performance computing center provide facilitator services to faculty for storage and compute. This includes free, distributed, and manageable storage services at a low level of size. If additional storage and compute are needed, consultations are arranged and fee-based solutions are offered to the researchers. The *research unit fee-for-service model* has three sustainable and flexible funding options, depending on the needs of the researcher: (1) a researcher uses a grant to pay the fees for storage, compute, and analytics and has complete access until the end of the award period; (2) a researcher pays a fee and his or her department supplements the fee, so that others in the department share the service and the researcher has access beyond the life of a grant; and (3) the campus pays 50 percent of the services, and faculty across campus can buy in. This model offers ways to distribute the costs differently, and can reduce costs across the research process, as researchers participate in evaluating trade-offs for services in out years. In the *all-campus coordination model*, there is a campus-wide committee: Policies, costs, and service boundaries are all shared, and transparency is paramount. The *institutional commitment model* requires a significant administrative investment into the library to provide research data management and a data repository. In one example, any student, staff, or faculty member has access to a private 100 GB of storage for 3 years and can publish up to 1 GB of data at no cost—these data will be available for a minimum of 10 years.

TABLE 5.1 Cooperative Approaches to Research Data Services

	Linked facilitator model	Research unit model	All-campus coordination model	Institutional commitment model
Motivation	Continuum of service	Sustainable, flexible shared cost models	Reduce stress and improve trust across units	Data life cycle as a driver
Service	Campus IT and local HPC Center provide information, "hand-off," and consulting	Storage and compute • 100% access (limited to award period) • Department pool/shared • Campus pool/50%	• Formalized Storage Council • Representatives from all units that provide storage • Awareness of policy changes	• All faculty, staff, and students • Private storage – 3 years 　◦ Longer with funding • Published data 　◦ Available 10 years 　◦ Increased allocation if funded
Benefit	• Range of "free" storage options on campus • Consulting • Infrastructure at scale	• Consultation • Genbank submissions • SysAdmin support	Cross-campus representatives to identify best storage solutions	• Data management plan support • Publishing support
Funding	Unfunded	Fee-for-service	Unit staff time	Administration; external project funding

NOTE: IT, information technology; HPC, high-performance computing.
SOURCE: Adapted from Melissa Cragin, San Diego Supercomputer Center, presentation to the workshop, July 12, 2019.

Cragin commented that Cornell University's library has developed an open-source web-based tool, Data Storage Finder, which can be customized for individual campuses. Faculty can use this tool to understand the storage services available on their respective campuses and to make better decisions. She explained that postsecondary institutions are beginning to recognize data as an asset: Campus-based cooperative arrangements are on the upswing; there is a trend toward professionalization of research staff roles; and an increased number of people and projects are being supported while managing costs. Persistent challenges include the variation of the kinds and extent of services across postsecondary institutions, hidden costs for data services across lifecycle and service groups, differences in procurement processes for multi-institution infrastructure projects that increase costs and necessitate much higher management overhead, and a lack of published empirical data on emergent trends and models.

Wendy Nilsen, NSF, explained that data are continuous, messy, and heterogeneous. Data are collected for long periods of time in large capacities, and biomedical data in particular can be combined to reveal important information about people. She described the success of the NSF-funded Asterisk database, which brings together data from diverse sources. Asterisk is now available on Apache and is being used by industry and researchers alike.

With the explosion of data, Nilsen noted the value of posing questions to data scientists and informaticians about what kind of data they need in order to move forward. She described a recent infrastructure initiative from NSF's Computer and Information Science and Engineering directorate to better understand the needs of the research community, including data that are usable, accessible, inexpensive, and machine-readable.

Nilsen's team considers how to develop infrastructure to collect and preserve relevant data. Questions to determine the relevance of data relate to quantity, reproducibility, cost (e.g., rare group samples are expensive), existence, and completeness. Her team evaluates analytics, crowdsourced value, diverse community governance, repetition, and feedback from users to determine the usefulness of data. She mentioned that 20 percent of NSF awards are now dedicated to outreach so that the researchers have the opportunity to get user feedback on their data. Expertise is also needed in computing and information science to reduce barriers to data access, maintain safety, increase data quality (e.g., metadata, validity, reproducibility), decrease costs (both time and money), and build sustainable models, she continued.

Lucy Ofiesh, Center for Open Science (COS), described the mission of COS as to increase openness, integrity, and reproducibility of research through three interconnected functions: infrastructure, metascience, and community (see Figure 5.2).

COS's metascience team studies the reproducibility of research, evaluates interventions, and works on large-scale reproduction projects. The technology team builds infrastructure, including several web-based solutions, that enables researchers to enact reproducible behaviors across the research life cycle. For example, OSF.io is a project management platform that has been implemented at 60 universities and research institutions across the world. Five million files were downloaded from OSF.io in 2018;

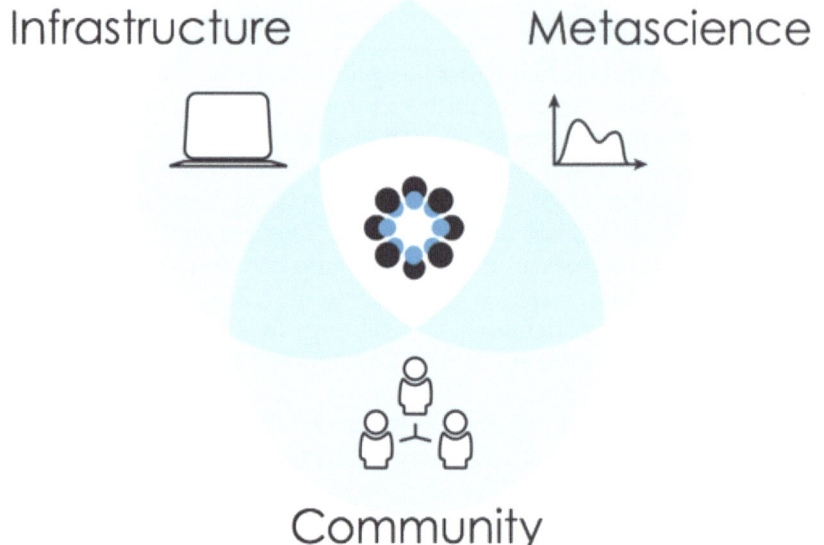

FIGURE 5.2 The mission of the Center for Open Science is reflected through three interconnected functions. SOURCE: Lucy Ofiesh, Center for Open Science, presentation to the workshop, July 12, 2019. Image available courtesy of CC-BY attribution license.

in 2019, that number climbed to nearly 12 million. She noted that OSF.io study registrations will likely be close to 40,000 by the close of 2019. People also use OSF.io to discover and repurpose files, papers, and data sets.

The community and policy team engages with existing research communities (and fosters new ones) to identify pain points in the research process and to develop best practices. The community and policy team is guided by eight transparency and openness guidelines:

1. Data citation,
2. Design transparency,
3. Research materials transparency,
4. Data transparency,
5. Analytic methods transparency,
6. Preregistration of studies,
7. Preregistration of analysis plans, and
8. Replication.

Data are multiplicatively more effective with open code, open materials, and preregistration of studies, Ofiesh explained. COS strives to motivate stakeholders, including publishers and funders, to recommend, require, and/or enforce sharing policies, which, with the help of technology solutions, will drive behavior change among members of the research community (see Figure 5.3).

Ofiesh emphasized that the first step to changing behavior is to understand the unique needs of each research community and develop relevant incentives. COS lends visibility to desired actions, thus promoting the adoption of ethical behavior. It is also exploring ways for researchers to earn credit, be acknowledged for their practice, and be viewed as credible (e.g., via the badging program for researchers who exhibit a best practice such as open data, open materials, or preregistration), as well as ways to support the use of open repositories and open registries. She noted that the proportion of preregistered open materials recently increased from 3 percent to 40 percent for the 60 journals that have adopted the badging program.

COS is also piloting programs related to registered reports, in which the researcher, journal, and funder are working together at the study design phase as well as engaging in peer review after both the study design phase and the report writing phase. This cooperative approach privileges rigorous scientific research and removes pressure for researchers to produce results that are "publishable." It also ensures that funders work in partnership with both the researcher and the journal throughout the research life cycle. Two hundred journals currently accept registered reports, Ofiesh said.

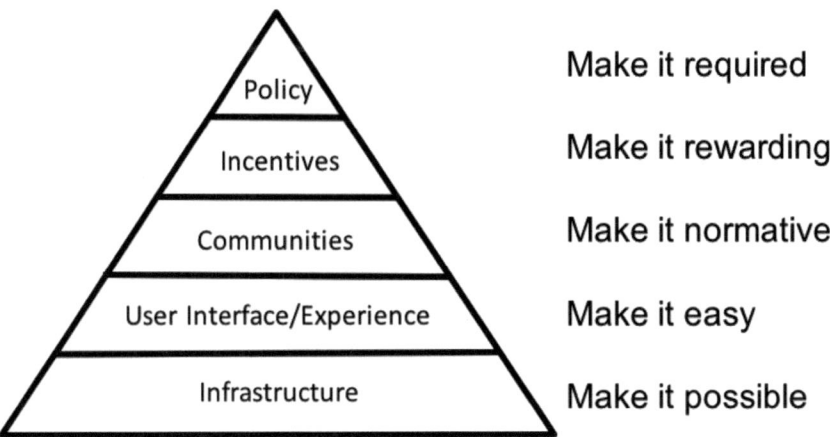

FIGURE 5.3 Key steps needed to change a research culture. SOURCE: Lucy Ofiesh, Center for Open Science, presentation to the workshop, July 12, 2019. Image available courtesy of CC-BY attribution license.

COS's long-term objectives are to (1) enable best practices with tools, communities, and policies; and (2) remain sustainable with technology solutions that ensure the security and duplicability of data. Ofiesh described a partnership between COS and Internet Archive to replicate all registrations on the COS website. This partnership provides an alternative to commercial infrastructure lock-in. COS strives to build products that meet researchers' needs, as those needs and the surrounding landscape continue to evolve.

Vilhuber observed that all four panelists emphasized that researchers are motivated by straightforward and inexpensive processes. However, it is difficult for postsecondary institutions to sustain such processes. He asked how to determine, from the researcher's perspective, which data are useful. Chodacki responded that this community's desire to solve all of the problems at once creates a multifaceted challenge. Instead, the community should figure out how to build systems to capture information consistently before making value judgments about data, he asserted. Cragin said that it is possible to determine the usefulness of some data with a long-tail perspective (i.e., thinking about integrated and interoperable data sets); but, there remains a need for theoretically based frameworks for decision making. Conversation about the implementation of standards and collection procedures is one way to engage with communities, although sectors within communities could have varied opinions (e.g., social scientists do not all share the same view of secondary uses of data). She added that it is important to think more broadly about data quality (e.g., the use of data for the public good versus the use of data at the institutional level). Nilsen agreed and said that it is crucial to understand what data are available and how they can be used. She reiterated that communities should share their experiences and pain points as a first step in eliminating barriers to data sharing. Ofiesh added that the adoption of any best practice begins with awareness, includes training, and results in refinement. If data are not shared, she cautioned, communities might miss opportunities to use data from other communities.

Maryann Martone, University of California, San Diego, asked Cragin whether the level of information technology support provided to research laboratories drives data management. She also wondered if disciplines have varied levels of interest in and need for such support. Cragin noted that the level of service offered varies by domain; for example, at Oregon State University's Center for Genome Research and Biocomputing, the high level of analytics support provided is attractive to and valuable for researchers. Chodacki echoed a comment from the first day of the workshop that research is inspired by creativity and curiosity. He noted an increased return on investment for the Carpentries and other training opportunities, which bring higher-level tools or skills into laboratories and feed this curiosity.

William Stead, Vanderbilt University Medical Center, asked about the cost to make Dryad freely available to all University of California researchers, and McCray wondered about the costs involved in COS's partnership with Internet Archive. Chodacki said that Dryad has an institutional membership model, with small ($3,000 per year), medium, and large ($13,000 per year) tiers. Ofiesh explained that the Institute of Museum and Library Services provided a 2-year $250,000 grant to build a connection to the COS application programming interface (API). Since Internet Archive is the lead on this project, COS is working with Internet Archives' API to push registries—a task that has the greatest cost. The cost to maintain the API is minimal; COS spends $200,000 a year to host and store data, but incremental costs over the long term will need to be supported.

In response to a question from Ilkay Altintas, University of California, San Diego, Cragin said that no good published research exists on the decision-making process to develop services and allocate resources across campus; most evidence is anecdotal. Altintas added that the definition of data is changing to include "services around data," which could change the cost model. Cragin clarified that her definition of services includes cyber infrastructure and software services and tools, which can be expensive to maintain, scale, and make interoperable. Robert Williams, University of Tennessee Health Science Center, explained that Dropbox has enabled a successful multi-institutional collaborative framework for data sharing. He described COS as an intermediary between Dropbox and Github, the latter of which is too complicated for use in his field. Chodacki observed that definitions of preservation also vary, further complicating the notion of forecasting costs for preservation. Adam Ferguson, University of California, San Francisco, pointed out that it is difficult to enforce data preservation policies on faculty who have 5-year grant cycles and little career stability. Sarah Nusser, Iowa State University, said that postsecondary institutions should be supporting preservation efforts regardless of faculty interest. Chodacki added that discussing how to forecast data preservation costs from a funder perspective is challenging, especially for cases in which the funder cannot allocate money for data preservation.

SUMMARIES OF SMALL-GROUP DISCUSSIONS

Connecting the Dots: Planning Tools for Data Support and Research Computing

Altintas said that her group discussed methods to encourage National Institutes of Health (NIH)-funded researchers to consider, update, and track lifetime data costs, although the group debated whether "lifetime" is the best way to describe what happens to data. She noted that training can be implemented to reduce costs and to motivate researchers. She suggested that training begin early (during scholarship) and be offered at the institutional level. She also proposed the adoption of a "train-the-trainers" model that follows existing practices, such as those used by the Carpentries. Another topic that emerged during the group's discussion was the need to align individual and institutional practices with expectations from federal agencies to develop economies of scale. The group also discussed cost reduction incentives embedded in new initiatives, such as NIH's Science and Technology Research Infrastructure for Discovery, Experimentation, and Sustainability.

Altintas explained that this community could learn lessons from other communities with decadal studies and best practices for planning. It is also imperative to define this community more precisely—who touches the data and when? She mentioned that existing methods to create reusable archives have not been standardized, and she noted the important difference (especially in terms of cost) between data preservation and data hoarding. One way to reduce the cost of data preservation is to make data inactive (i.e., suspended animation or "dehydrated" data). This requires little energy and ensures that the data have captured knowledge and are findable. An inactive archive could then be refreshed at a low cost to improve the value of the data and to prevent loss. Another way to reduce cost is to create an ecosystem of universities and national funding agencies that could distribute the responsibilities to support the operation of repositories, she continued. A related problem that needs to be addressed is that funding for data generation does not always align with funding for data acceptance; thus, repositories are responsible for finding creative ways to reduce the cost of their operations in order to accept more data.

Practices for Using Biomedical Data Knowledge Networks for Life-cycle Cost Forecasting and Updating

Clifford Lynch, Coalition for Networked Information, said that his group first tried to develop an understanding of the phrase "biomedical data knowledge networks." The group framed its understanding of this concept in terms of the complex and important connection between (1) communities that work with classes of data; and (2) platforms that store, analyze, preserve, and share data for communities. The group discussed several ways to mobilize and leverage communities and platforms to help with cost forecasting. Because these communities are powerful engines for developing standards and establishing practices and norms, he noted that they could predict expected production rates from instrumentation. Lynch explained that in order to forecast access and preservation costs, it is crucial to understand the extent to which access and preservation encompass the platforms themselves—in other words, what is the life span of platforms before the data go into "hibernation"?

He noted that the best platforms (i.e., the ones that provide incentives and build and strengthen the community) are not passive places for storing and taking data. Rather, they are environments that actively improve and add value to data as well as offer tools to analyze and compare data. Lynch explained that tools in a common environment provide benchmarks against which progress in the field can be measured. He noted that the group considered how to move resources that have risen to a certain level of importance into a more stable, long-term funding cycle. The group also discussed the need for governance of these platforms as well as the need to better understand the relationships between platforms and journals. In response to a topic raised by the previous group, Lynch's group noted that scholarly societies could play a role in helping to codify membership in this "community."

Incentivizing Researchers to Determine the Costs of Interoperability

Charles Manski, Northwestern University, explained that several members of his group defined interoperability as the "production-level dissemination" of research. He noted that issues of semantics illustrate the divide between the data community and the research community. For example, he said that many researchers do not use the term "interoperability" or the acronym "FAIR." With different uses of language, communication between the two groups can become more difficult, he continued.

Manski shared a series of comments made by group members. One participant said that data scientists should be engaged at the start of the research process to assist with dissemination and data sharing. Another participant said that it is difficult to ask researchers to comply with ever-changing specifications for making data available. Researchers are not funded for such activities, and, with the continual change, the process loses value and more closely resembles bureaucracy. Another participant suggested that scientific papers should make science interoperable. The group also discussed ways to incentivize researchers to see that data have value; perhaps the onus should be on the postsecondary institutions, not the researchers, to generate the data, Manski explained. Lastly, the group discussed the sharing of clinical data: Some group members thought that doing so violates patient privacy, while others thought that privacy was simply a mask for data blocking and territoriality.

6

Reflections and Next Steps

PANEL DISCUSSION: RESEARCHERS' PERSPECTIVES ON NEXT STEPS

Margaret Levenstein, University of Michigan, Moderator
Nuno Bandeira, University of California, San Diego
Jessie Tenenbaum, Duke University and the North Carolina Department of Health and Human Services
Georgia (Gina) Tourassi, Oak Ridge National Laboratory
Robert Williams, University of Tennessee Health Science Center

Margaret Levenstein, University of Michigan, invited the research community representatives who shared their perspectives on the first day of the workshop (see Chapter 2) to participate in the final panel discussion of the workshop. She asked the researchers to reflect on the following questions, based on the information that was shared over the course of the workshop:

- What are your needs, and what could you use to reduce the costs of sharing, preserving, and providing access to data over the data life cycle?
- What incentives (both positive and negative) would reduce costs and encourage researchers to share their data?
- What tools and practices could the National Library of Medicine (NLM) use to help researchers to better integrate risk management

practices and considerations into data preservation, archiving, and accessing decisions?
- What methods would encourage National Institutes of Health (NIH)-funded researchers to consider, update, and track lifetime data costs? How do researchers make decisions that will affect their costs, the costs of data, and the quality and accessibility of data throughout the data life cycle?
- How do we address the burdens on academic researchers and industry staff to implement these tools, methods, and practices?

Robert Williams, University of Tennessee Health Science Center, observed that the first day of the workshop was focused primarily on the preservation and curation of *human data*. He reiterated that there is important work in long-tail animal modeling and noted that the National Institute on Drug Abuse provides $250 million each year for rat research. However, almost none of those data are integrated in any kind of uniform database and thus are not linkable. He said that resources need to be built to allow investigators to link their data effectively. He suggested educating investigators early and giving them tools that will automatically connect data. During the past 20 years, Williams has been building families of genetically diverse animals that can be used to compute correlation coefficients. Such work relies on multiplicity—some data should be available forever, and thus "life cycle" is the wrong phrase to use to describe data. He reiterated a concern that surfaced multiple times throughout the workshop about how to determine which data are valuable. He suggested that data are valuable (and should be kept) if they are linkable, usable, and able to "breathe and breed."

Georgia (Gina) Tourassi, Oak Ridge National Laboratory, emphasized that data, algorithms, and code will continue to be produced at a speed faster than that of policy and regulation. She said that it is difficult to forecast lifetime costs and risks because the definition of "valuable data sets" will change over time. Considering the differences across application domains, it is clear that a one-size-fits-all approach does not work, she asserted. Costs and risks will depend on storage, computations, and the number of users accessing the resources. Moving forward, she suggested a two-pronged approach: Academic researchers will always be limited by the lifetime of their grants and their funding, so it is unfair to ask them to make scientific advances *and* to deploy data sets, algorithms, and software in formats that are of operational value. Instead, she continued, the scientific community should develop policies for best practices. At the end of the funding cycle, when data have become a federal asset, they could move to an entity (e.g., a federal coordinated infrastructure) that would be responsible for the lifetime management of the data. She noted that funding and well-defined metrics are needed to establish the value of different data sets, benchmark algorithms, and maintain transparencies and reproducibility. She suggested increased funding for algorithms as well as for techniques for data privacy and data curation, which could help change the culture of the scientific community. Statistical methods are also needed to determine whether a synthetic data set is reliable. Lastly, because data science is infused across all disciplines, she noted a need for more undergraduate and graduate training programs on best practices.

Jessie Tenenbaum, Duke University and the North Carolina Department of Health and Human Services, emphasized Butte's and Tourassi's assertions that requests for applications for data reuse and for curation tools and approaches would be very helpful. Because there are so many ways to integrate data, she noted that it could be interesting to write a review paper about the many different approaches that people use to integrate data. This could lead to a better understanding of the technical requirements for how data are shared. She championed the notion of improving education and changing the culture instead of forcing researchers with "carrots and sticks," as well as involving all stakeholders from the start of the research process. She concluded by suggesting that researchers aim for conducting *translucent* research instead of *transparent* research, especially when working with clinical data.

Nuno Bandeira, University of California, San Diego, said that a discussion about data preservation should include the costs of data reutilization: If data are not going to be reused, why pay to store them? He added that data need to be interoperable—integrated with tools, workflows, compute resources, and community-scale tools for meta-analysis. He suggested evaluating the "data community cost" instead of the "data storage cost." Although he applauded the postsecondary institutions that recognize the value of data and have allocated resources accordingly toward preservation, he worried that it will be difficult to create a community around data if standards for data preservation are not uniform across institutions and data types. He provided a cautionary tale about the first proteomics mass spectrometry repository effort, which failed because it was a federated system (i.e., the responsibility for storing data was distributed to various institutions). He emphasized the need for stewards in the data community (i.e., people who are responsible for determining community needs; building standards; communicating; and promoting data persistence, interoperability, and reusability). Those entities are currently called repositories, but Bandeira and Clifford Lynch, Coalition for Networked Information, proposed using the term "platforms" instead. Bandeira noted that the additional cost of such an entity needs to be considered in conversations about data preservation. He closed by emphasizing that even though it is important to organize data communities, their members should not have to provide for their own compute and storage capabilities.

Levenstein highlighted the panelists' focus on "community" and the cost to create and maintain such a community around data, which is different from the cost to preserve data. She noted the panelists' interest in creating a repository community, in particular. Repositories, like researchers, need to be trained to prepare and preserve data as well as to understand what standards exist across other repositories, she continued. These actions create "stewardship." Although these changes may not reduce cost, she emphasized that these actions will increase the value of what is preserved.

Williams suggested developing a funding mechanism that would enable the interoperability of research efforts, and Levenstein mentioned an organization of repositories in the social sciences and statistical communities called Data-PASS.[1] She added that the Research Data Alliance has also tried to create a community. Patricia Flatley Brennan, NLM, explained that NLM would like to increase the efficiency of spending and decrease waste rather than simply cut costs. She appreciated Tourassi's statement that NLM has a federal asset, which society deserves to have fully utilized. Brennan said that NIH recognizes the need for enterprise-level solutions as well as institute-specific solutions, which complicates the "community approach"—many communities do not align directly with any single institute or center in NIH. She reiterated her request to the National Academies' study committee to help NLM think about the preservation of existing data as well as preparation for the preservation of future data. She appreciated the participants' comments about the importance of helping new investigators to understand, at the start of their training, what it means to create a data strategy that focuses on future interoperability. She hopes that this committee's work might inspire the scientific communities to take on the difficult task of providing metrics for data value. Levenstein reiterated the suggestion for NIH to develop funding mechanisms for data preservation, data curation, and secondary use of data. She also reiterated the suggestion to require a section in proposals for prior data collection. Brennan mentioned an NLM initiative to fund computational approaches to curation. NIH plans on soon releasing a separate research-resource funding mechanism. Philip Bourne, University of Virginia, expressed his support for such a mechanism and noted that certain constraints related to data governance should appear in the requests for applications, which would allow greater integration across different resources as they evolve.

Lars Vilhuber, Cornell University, said that early career training for researchers (e.g., tools to think about data, methods to self-curate data,

---

[1] For more information about Data-PASS, see http://data-pass.org, accessed September 25, 2019.

strategies to integrate platforms) is critical. The goal is not to transform researchers into data curators or programmers but rather to raise their awareness of possible solutions to problems. He mentioned the Registry of Research Data Repositories,[2] which is a *database* of repositories, not a *community* of repositories. Although it has not been actively maintained, it has elements that could be leveraged to serve and build communities. Monica McCormick, University of Delaware Library, suggested that librarians and other partners in the research process should also be eligible for funded training. Warren Kibbe, Duke University, expressed his support for a separate research-resource funding mechanism but requested that it include awards for 7 years instead of for 5 years. Bandeira pointed out that some journals require a 10-year period for the persistence of the data, which extends beyond any current funding mechanism. Kibbe suggested that the process for building a community and engaging that community in the operation of a resource needs to be codified, which relates to the governance of each resource. He referenced a recent proposal to the National Cancer Institute to ensure that data management plans and data sharing plans are included in every submission. This will allow researchers to prepare to disseminate information, preserve data, and make data available for reuse in the future.

THEMES AND OPPORTUNITIES

Several important themes and opportunities were raised during the workshop presentation and discussions, including the following:

- *The nature of research is changing.* The distinction between data contributors and data users is blurring as research becomes increasingly data-driven (Brennan). Researchers need to consider the entire life cycle of research, from the conception of an idea, spanning the final publication, and including any data reuse that may occur afterward (Vilhuber). Data management plans can help (John Chodacki, University of California Curation Center, California Digital Library). The next generation of researchers will need crosscutting skill sets (Bourne). Expertise in computing and information science can lessen barriers to data access, help maintain safety, increase data quality, and decrease costs (Wendy Nilsen, National Science Foundation). With this shift, it becomes even more important for researchers, funders, and other

---

[2] For more information about the Registry of Research Data Repositories, see http://re3data.org, accessed September 25, 2019.

stakeholders to be able to estimate long-term data costs so they can plan accordingly (Brennan).
- *Research culture needs to evolve.* Approaches to increase FAIR—findable, accessible, interoperable, reusable—data may help expand the types of data that are available to researchers and increase the return on research investments (Adam Ferguson, University of California, San Francisco). However, cultural changes are needed to expand data curation and data sharing efforts (Levenstein). Developing domain-specific standards to determine what constitutes high-quality data could help (Bandeira), as could the development of more user-friendly interfaces and tools that support visualization, discoverability, and cost estimation (Tenenbaum). Tools are also needed to make it easier for researchers to curate data during the research process. Potential changes to the grant process could also help, perhaps by encouraging researchers to disclose any prior data that they had collected in addition to the prior research that they had conducted (Levenstein's subgroup). Academic institutions could also become more involved in motivating researchers to share data (Atul Butte, University of California, San Francisco). An important first step in changing behavior is to understand the unique needs of each research community and develop relevant incentives (Lucy Ofiesh, Center for Open Science). Additional training offered early and throughout a researcher's career could improve adoption (subgroup led by Ilkay Altintas, University of California, San Diego).
- *Stakeholders' roles are changing.* Bourne indicated that it is important to consider the changing roles of various data stakeholders, including funders, researchers, resource developers, publishers, literature readers and authors, academic administrators, faculty, and students. The current ecosystem is evolving. For example, while some publishers are currently requiring that data be deposited into a repository in order to publish the results, it is unclear if these repositories will be reliable or sustainable. Academic approaches toward data also need to change to ensure that they can train data professionals, use academic data to improve productivity, improve data infrastructure, bolster academic libraries as they transition from data preservationists to data analysts, and update institutional data policies (Bourne). It is important that preservation policies and plans to make data accessible and reusable over time move from being ad hoc processes to being openly discussed and planned for among relevant stakeholders (Chodacki).

- *Data use agreements are important.* Amy O'Hara, Georgetown University, explained that data use agreements can help manage the financial, legal, social, and emotional risks associated with acquiring, managing, and curating data. While these agreements can codify terms and conditions to ensure that each party interacts with the data responsibly, the terms of use have to be clear, especially regarding subsequent data use, and an authority has to be defined who will approve and explain the agreement and foster continued responsible use of the data (O'Hara).
- *Ensuring long-term access to digital content is crucial.* Trevor Owens, U.S. Library of Congress, illustrated the National Digital Stewardship Alliance's five risk areas for planning and policy development for digital preservation—storage and geographic location of the data, file fixity and data integrity, information security, metadata, and file formats. These risks might be best mitigated by having a permanent trained staff working in these areas and planning for a continual refresh cycle of software and hardware (Owens).
- *Privacy concerns need to be balanced with research goals.* Brad Malin, Vanderbilt University Medical Center, raised multiple privacy-preserving frameworks, including data deidentification, encrypted computations, secure hardware, and blockchain approaches. However, none of these will address all privacy concerns. Thus, it is important to determine an appropriate level of risk and to ensure accountability in a system (Malin). Universities and research communities have important roles in implementing privacy models (e.g., tiered models or improved consent templates) and better applying privacy preserving techniques to data (Vilhuber's subgroup).
- *Infrastructure investments can help.* Data platforms are often not equipped to handle the volume, velocity, and variety of data that researchers would like to apply to emerging research questions (Ferguson). Resources need to be built to allow researchers to link their data effectively (Williams). The value of data increases as they are integrated with other data (Alexa McCray, Harvard Medical Center) and can be more effective when paired with open code, open materials, and preregistration of studies (Ofiesh). Sustained infrastructure investments could help advance scientific discovery (Tourassi). However, the costs associated with building and maintaining relevant platforms should be factored into data access and preservation costs; it is important to understand the life span of a platform and plan for its governance and ultimate

transition (subgroup led by Clifford Lynch, Coalition for Networked Information).
- *Risks and costs of research data in the cloud need to be considered.* The subgroup led by David Maier, Portland State University, discussed that once data have been collected and stored with a cloud provider, new costs and risks emerge. For example, egress costs accrue from users accessing the data and these costs need to be planned for. Some states and municipal governments have preferred cloud providers, which can inhibit the use of other providers. Also, certain mechanisms and restrictions that have been placed on the data may not effectively transfer to cloud-enabled computing and storage. These and other considerations need to be thought through during the decision-making process for cloud storage (Maier's subgroup).
- *Access to and use of active data needs to be facilitated.* Melissa Cragin, San Diego Supercomputer Center, described four different models to support research data services, including the unfunded linked facilitator model, the research unit fee-for-service model, the all campus coordination model, and the institutional commitment model. Each has its own benefits, challenges, and limitations. Sustainable models are needed (Cragin).

Bourne mentioned an issue that had not been discussed during the workshop: the value of data coordination centers and the role that they play in preservation. Maryann Martone, University of California, San Diego, agreed and noted that the data ecosystem (i.e., where data are, who is responsible for them, who has access to them) remains broad and includes many ongoing efforts. She championed the value of creating a PubMed-like infrastructure for data. She added that more data are needed to understand the number of institutional repositories that already exist. This broad and complex problem speaks to the data problem itself, she continued. The notion of a one-size-fits-all solution is intractable because data are generated in so many places and for so many different uses. She added that despite numerous efforts to establish catalogues over the past 10 years, many people remain unaware of their existence. Many members of the research community spend their time in the laboratory or the field and might not be aware of the resources available to them online. She also described the diverse skill sets in the research community that should be appreciated and utilized. She explained that the system needs to be managed in such a way that every researcher can reach his or her maximum value and then facilitate a future hand-off to the person with the right expertise for the next step in the process.

Martone commented that effective data management in the laboratory is essential for data sharing. The use of standards in the laboratory could facilitate data sharing and curation; however, data sharing could also facilitate the development of standards. She explained that barriers to entry will always exist; however, more needs to be understood about how standards and tools could lower costs and other barriers. She said that working with data is rarely simple or inexpensive, and, at the moment, many researchers do not value long-term preservation of data beyond the research life cycle. She appreciated Williams' comments about animal research to highlight how different the data problems are in each domain. Large, rich, public data sets that enable discovery are important, and new methods can allow access to old data; however, long-term costs are unknown, she continued.

Martone said that incentives are not homogeneous. "Carrots and sticks" often work in tandem, and a mandate could be useful to initiate data sharing. However, to maintain data sharing, there needs to be value for the researcher beyond the mandate. She emphasized that early training is essential for researchers, as is institutional funding for repositories. Partnerships with libraries have been especially fruitful—guiding researchers to resources and providing expertise about data management and preservation.

Martone emphasized that efforts in data preservation and scientific discovery have to be synchronized. This workshop reiterated that this process is expensive and difficult, but it also highlighted the larger issue, which is that inefficiency exists throughout the system. Greater understanding is needed as to how individuals' practices are impacted by infrastructure, she continued. For example, some researchers store copies of their data in addition to storing the data in a repository. Martone highlighted a previous point made by Cragin that although large grants are given for instruments, the data infrastructure that is required to handle data that emerge from these instruments is drastically underestimated. Martone also highlighted the absence of a good understanding of how much money from each grant is being allocated for data preparation and curation; likely, the costs are higher than realized. Liability costs are also of critical importance to avoid lawsuits.

In closing the workshop, Martone emphasized that communities are ready to use the wealth of existing tools and expertise available to think seriously about data management. However, funding mechanisms to create platforms to connect expertise and allow people to share experiences are still needed. McCray thanked participants for increasing the value of the workshop for the committee's study and for the broader community.

References

Chakradhar, S. 2017. Predictable response: Finding optimal drugs and doses using artificial intelligence. *Nature Medicine* 23(11):1244-1247.

Ioannidis, J.P.A. 2005. Why most published research findings are false. *PLoS Med* 2(8):e124.

Macleod, M.R., S. Michie, I. Roberts, U. Dirnagl, I. Chalmers, J.P.A. Ioannidis, R. Al-Shahi Salman, A.-W. Chan, and P. Glasziou. 2014. Biomedical research: Increasing value, reducing waste. *The Lancet* 383(9912):101-104.

Neff, E.P. 2018. Dark data see the light. *LabAnimal* 47(2):45-48.

Nielson, J., J. Paquette, A.W. Liu, C.F. Guandique, C.A. Tovar, T. Inoue, K.-A. Irvine, et al. 2015. Topological data analysis for discovery in preclinical spinal cord injury and traumatic brain injury. *Nature Communications* 6:8581.

Phillips, M., J. Bailey, A. Goethals, and T. Owens. 2013. The NDSA Levels of Digital Preservation: An explanation and uses. Pp. 216-222 in *Proceedings of the 2013 IS&T Archiving Conference*. Society for Imaging Science and Technology. https://www.imaging.org/site/ist.

Wilkinson, M.D., M. Dumontier, I.J. Aalbersberg, G. Appleton, M. Axton, A. Baak, and N. Blomberg, et al. 2016. The FAIR guiding principles for scientific data management and stewardship. *Scientific Data* 3:160018.

Appendixes

A

Workshop Agenda

National Academy of Sciences Building
Washington, DC

Thursday, July 11, 2019

8:30 a.m.	**Welcome and Introductory Remarks**
	David Chu, Institute for Defense Analyses,
	    Study Committee Chair
	Tyler Kloefkorn, National Academies of Sciences,
	    Engineering, and Medicine
	Sammantha Magsino, National Academies

8:45	**Sponsor Expectations** Patricia Flatley Brennan, National Library of Medicine
9:00	**The Burdens and Benefits of "Long-Tail" Data Sharing** Adam Ferguson, University of California, San Francisco
10:00	Break
10:20	**Panel Discussion: Researchers' Perspectives—Managing Risks and Forecasting Costs for Long-Term Data Preservation**

          Moderator: Margaret Levenstein, University of Michigan, Study Committee Member

Panelists:
Nuno Bandeira, University of California, San Diego
Jessie Tenenbaum, Duke University, North Carolina
    Department of Health and Human Services
Georgia Tourassi, Oak Ridge National Laboratory
Robert Williams, University of Tennessee Health Science Center

11:40	**Panel Discussion: Addressing Data Risks and Their Costs** Moderator: Michelle Meyer, Geisinger, Study Committee Member *Panelists:* Amy O'Hara, Georgetown University Brad Malin, Vanderbilt University Medical Center Trevor Owens, U.S. Library of Congress
12:40 p.m.	Lunch
1:30	**Breakout Sessions—Tools and Practices That NLM Could Use to Help Researchers and Funders Better Integrate Risk Management Practices and Considerations into Data Preservation, Archiving, and Accessing Decisions**

Session 1-A Mechanisms for Forecasting the Costs of Maintained Privacy	Session 1-B Mechanisms for Identifying Risk and Cost Factors of Research Data in the Cloud	Session 1-C Mechanisms for Identifying the Costs of Making Data Truly Findable
Moderator: Michelle Meyer Rapporteur: Lars Vilhuber	Moderator: Dave Maier Rapporteur: Ilkay Altintas	Moderator: Bill Stead Rapporteur: Maggie Levenstein

2:30	Break
2:45	**Report on Breakout Sessions**

APPENDIX A 65

3:00	**Data—What's It Going to Cost and What's in It for Me?** Philip Bourne, University of Virginia
4:00	**Precisely Practicing Medicine from 700 Trillion Points of Data** Atul Butte, University of California, San Francisco [participating remotely]
4:45	**Open Discussion—Reflections, Plans for Day 2, Coordination with Study** Alexa McCray, Harvard Medical School, Study Committee Member
5:15	Adjourn for the Day

Friday, July 12, 2019

8:30 a.m.	**Introductory Remarks** Alexa McCray, Harvard Medical School, Study Committee Member
8:40	**Panel Discussion: Incentives, Mechanisms, and Practices for Improved Awareness of Cost Consequences in Data Decisions** Moderator: Lars Vilhuber, Cornell University, Study Committee Member *Panelists:* *John Chodacki, University of California Curation Center, California Digital Library* *Melissa Cragin, San Diego Supercomputer Center* *Wendy Nilsen, National Science Foundation* *Lucy Ofiesh, Center for Open Science*
10:00	**Breakout Sessions—Methods to Encourage NIH-funded Researchers to Consider, Update, and Track Lifetime Data Costs**

Session 2-A	Session 2-B	Session 2-C
Connecting the Dots: Planning Tools for Data Support and Research Computing	Practices for Using Biomedical Data Knowledge Networks for Life-cycle Cost Forecasting and Updating	Incentivizing Researchers to Determine the Costs of Interoperability
Moderator: Ilkay Altintas Rapporteur: Dave Maier	Moderator: Cliff Lynch Rapporteur: Lars Vilhuber	Moderator: Bill Stead Rapporteur: Chuck Manski

11:00 Break

11:15 **Report on Breakout Sessions**

11:30 **Panel Discussion: Researchers' Perspectives—Reflections and Next Steps**
Moderator: Margaret Levenstein, University of Michigan, Study Committee Member

Panelists:
Nuno Bandeira, University of California, San Diego
Jessie Tenenbaum, Duke University, North Carolina Department of Health and Human Services
Georgia Tourassi, Oak Ridge National Laboratory
Robert Williams, University of Tennessee Health Science Center

12:20 p.m. **Closing Remarks—Themes and Opportunities**
Maryann Martone, University of California, San Diego; Study Committee Member

12:30 Adjourn Workshop

B

Biographical Sketches of Committee

DAVID S.C. CHU, *Chair*, serves as president of the Institute for Defense Analyses (IDA). IDA is a nonprofit corporation operating in the public interest. Its three federally funded research and development centers provide objective analyses of national security issues and related national challenges, particularly those requiring extraordinary scientific and technical expertise. As president, Dr. Chu directs the activities of more than 1,000 scientists and technologists. Together, they conduct and support research requested by federal agencies involved in advancing national security and advising on science and technology issues. Dr. Chu served in the Department of Defense (DoD) as Under Secretary of Defense for Personnel and Readiness from 2001–2009 and earlier as Assistant Secretary of Defense and Director for Program Analysis and Evaluation from 1981–1993. From 1978–1981, he was the assistant director of the Congressional Budget Office for National Security and International Affairs. Dr. Chu served in the U. S. Army from 1968–1970. He was an economist with the RAND Corporation from 1970–1978, director of RAND's Washington Office from 1994–1998, and vice president for its Army Research Division from 1998–2001. He earned his doctorate in economics, as well as a bachelor of arts in economics and mathematics, from Yale University. Dr. Chu is a member of the Defense Science Board and a fellow of the National Academy of Public Administration (NAPA). He is a recipient of the DoD Medal for Distinguished Public Service with Gold Palm, the Department of Veterans Affairs Meritorious Service Award, the Department of the Army Distinguished Civilian Service Award, the Department of the Navy

Distinguished Public Service Award, and the NAPA's National Public Service Award.

ILKAY ALTINTAS is the chief data science officer at the San Diego Supercomputer Center (SDSC), University of California, San Diego (UCSD), where she is also the founder and director for the Workflows for Data Science Center of Excellence, and a fellow of the Halicioglu Data Science Institute. In her various roles and projects, she leads collaborative multidisciplinary teams with a research objective to deliver impactful results through making computational data science work more reusable, programmable, scalable, and reproducible. Since joining SDSC in 2001, she has been a principal investigator (PI) and a technical leader in a wide range of cross-disciplinary projects. Her work has been applied to many scientific and societal domains including bioinformatics, geoinformatics, high-energy physics, multiscale biomedical science, smart cities, and smart manufacturing. She is a co-initiator of the popular open-source Kepler Scientific Workflow System and the co-author of publications related to computational data science at the intersection of workflows, provenance, distributed computing, big data, reproducibility, and software modeling in many different application areas. Among the awards she has received are the 2015 Institute of Electrical and Electronics Engineers (IEEE) Technical Committee on Scalable Computing Award for Excellence in Scalable Computing for Early Career Researchers and the 2017 Association for Computing Machinery (ACM) Special Interest Group on High Performance Computing's Emerging Woman Leader in Technical Computing Award.

GOLAM SAYEED CHOUDHURY is the associate dean for research data management and Hodson Director of the Digital Research and Curation Center at the Sheridan Libraries of Johns Hopkins University. Choudhury is also a member of the executive committee for the Institute of Data Intensive Engineering and Science based at Johns Hopkins University. Dr. Choudhury is a President Obama appointee to the National Museum and Library Services Board. He was a member of the National Academies of Sciences, Engineering, and Medicine's Board on Research Data and Information and the Blue Ribbon Task Force on Sustainable Digital Preservation and Access. He has testified for the Research Subcommittee of the Committee on Science, Space, and Technology. He was a member of the board of the National Information Standards Organization, OpenAIRE2020, DuraSpace, the Inter-university Consortium for Political and Social Research (ICPSR) Council, Digital Library Federation Advisory Committee, Library of Congress' National Digital Stewardship Alliance Coordinating Committee, Federation of Earth Scientists Information

APPENDIX B   69

Partnership Executive Committee, and the Project MUSE Advisory Board. Dr. Choudhury was a member of the EDUCAUSE Center for Analysis and Research Data Curation Working Group. He has been a senior presidential fellow with the Council on Library and Information Resources, a lecturer in the Department of Computer Science at Johns Hopkins and a research fellow at the Graduate School of Library and Information Science at the University of Illinois, Urbana-Champaign. He is the recipient of the 2012 Online Computer Library Center, Incorporated/Library and Information Technology Association Kilgour Award. Dr. Choudhury has served as PI for projects funded through the National Science Foundation (NSF), Institute of Museum and Library Services, Library of Congress' NDIIPP, Alfred P. Sloan Foundation, Andrew W. Mellon Foundation, Microsoft Research, and a Maryland-based venture capital group. He is the product owner for the Data Conservancy, which focuses on the development of data curation infrastructure, and the Public Access Submission System, which supports simultaneous submission of articles to PubMed Central and institutional repositories. He has oversight for data curation research and development and data archive implementation at the Sheridan Libraries at Johns Hopkins University. Dr. Choudhury has published articles in journals such as the *International Journal of Digital Curation*, *D-Lib*, the *Journal of Digital Information*, *First Monday*, and *Library Trends*. He has served on committees for the Digital Curation Conference, Open Repositories, Joint Conference on Digital Libraries, and Web-Wise. He has presented at various conferences including EDUCAUSE, the Coalition for Networked Information, Jisc-Coalition for Networked Information, Digital Library Federation, American Library Association, Association of College and Research Libraries, and international venues including the International Federation of Library Associations and Institutions, the Kanazawa Information Technology Roundtable, eResearch Australasia, the North America-China Conference, eResearch New Zealand, and the Arabian-Gulf Chapter of the Special Libraries Conference.

MARGARET LEVENSTEIN is director of ICPSR; research professor at the Institute for Social Research and the School of Information; and adjunct professor of business economics and public policy at the Stephen M. Ross School of Business. She has taught economics at the University of Michigan since 1990. She serves as co-executive director of the Michigan Federal Statistical Research Data Center (FSRDC) and co-chair of the Executive Committee of the FSRDC national network. She is the associate chair of the American Economic Association's Committee on the Status of Women in the Economics Profession and past president of the Business History Conference. She is PI of CenHRS, a Sloan Foundation-funded project building an enhancement to the Health and Retirement Study based on linkages to administrative and survey data on Health and Retirement Study employers and co-workers. She is PI of an NSF-funded project to establish a repository of linked data and data linkage algorithms at ICPSR; a Sloan and NSF-funded effort to establish a Researcher Passport using open badges for credentialed, trusted researchers to access restricted data; and an NSF-funded project conducting experiments to encourage citizen-scientists to improve research metadata. She received a Ph.D. in economics from Yale University and a B.A. from Barnard College, Columbia University. She is the author of numerous studies on competition and collusion, the development of information systems, and using "organic" data to improve social and economic measurement.

CLIFFORD LYNCH has been the executive director of the Coalition for Networked Information (CNI) since 1997. CNI, jointly sponsored by the Association of Research Libraries and EDUCAUSE, includes about 200 member organizations concerned with the intelligent uses of information technology and networked information to enhance scholarship and intellectual life. CNI's wide-ranging agenda includes work in digital preservation, data intensive scholarship, teaching, learning and technology, and infrastructure and standards development. Prior to joining CNI, Dr. Lynch spent 18 years at the University of California Office of the President, the last 10 as director of library automation. Dr. Lynch, who holds a Ph.D. in computer science from the University of California, Berkeley, is an adjunct professor at Berkeley's School of Information. He is both a past president and recipient of the Award of Merit of the American Society for Information Science and a fellow of the American Association for the Advancement of Science, the ACM, and the National Information Standards Organization. He served as co-chair of the National Academies' Board on Research Data and Information from 2011–2016; he is active on numerous advisory boards and visiting committees. His work has been recognized by the American Library Association's Lippincott Award, the EDUCAUSE Leadership Award in Public Policy and Practice, and the American Society for Engineering Education's Homer Bernhardt Award.

DAVID MAIER is Maseeh Professor of Emerging Technologies at Portland State University. Prior to his current position, he was on the faculty at the State University of New York, Stony Brook, and Oregon Graduate Institute. He has spent extended visits with Inria, the University of Wisconsin, Madison, Microsoft Research, and the National University of Singapore. He is the author of books on relational databases, logic programming, and object-oriented databases, as well as papers on database theory, object-oriented technology, scientific databases, and dataspace management. He is a recognized expert on the challenges of large-scale data in the sciences.

He received an NSF Young Investigator Award in 1984 and was awarded the 1997 ACM Special Interest Group on Management of Data's Innovations Award for his contributions in objects and databases. He is also an ACM Fellow and IEEE Senior Member. He holds a dual B.A. in mathematics and in computer science from the University of Oregon (Honors College, 1974) and a Ph.D. in electrical engineering and computer science from Princeton University (1978).

CHARLES MANSKI has been Board of Trustees Professor in Economics at Northwestern University since 1997. He previously was a faculty member at the University of Wisconsin, Madison (1983–1998), the Hebrew University of Jerusalem (1979–1983), and Carnegie Mellon University (1973–1980). He received his B.S. and Ph.D. in economics from the Massachusetts Institute of Technology (MIT) in 1970 and 1973, respectively. He has received honorary doctorates from the University of Rome 'Tor Vergata' (2006) and the Hebrew University of Jerusalem (2018). Dr. Manski's research spans econometrics, judgment and decision, and analysis of public policy. He is author of *Public Policy in an Uncertain World* (Harvard 2013), *Identification for Prediction and Decision* (Harvard 2007), *Social Choice with Partial Knowledge of Treatment Response* (Princeton 2005), *Partial Identification of Probability Distributions* (Springer 2003), *Identification Problems in the Social Sciences* (Harvard 1995), and *Analog Estimation Methods in Econometrics* (Chapman & Hall 1988); co-author of *College Choice in America* (Harvard 1983); and co-editor of *Evaluating Welfare and Training Programs* (Harvard 1992) and *Structural Analysis of Discrete Data with Econometric Applications* (MIT 1981). He has served as director of the Institute for Research on Poverty (1988–1991), chair of the Board of Overseers of the Panel Study of Income Dynamics (1994–1998), and chair of the National Academies Committee on Data and Research for Policy on Illegal Drugs (1998–2001). Editorial service includes terms as editor of the *Journal of Human Resources* (1991–1994), co-editor of the *Econometric Society Monograph Series* (1983–1988), member of the editorial board of the *Annual Review of Economics* (2007–2013), member of the Report Review Committee of the National Academies (2010–2018), and associate editor of the *Annals of Applied Statistics* (2006–2010), *Econometrica*, (1980–1988), *Journal of Economic Perspectives* (1986–1989), *Journal of the American Statistical Association* (1983–1985, 2002–2004), and *Transportation Science* (1978–1984). Dr. Manski is an elected member of the National Academy of Sciences. He is an elected fellow of the American Academy of Arts and Sciences, the Econometric Society, the American Statistical Association, and the American Association for the Advancement of Science, distinguished fellow of the American Economic Association, and corresponding fellow of the British Academy.

MARYANN MARTONE is a professor emerita at UCSD but still maintains an active laboratory and currently serves as the chair of the University of California Academic Senate Committee on Academic Computing and Communications. She received her B.A. from Wellesley College in biological psychology and ancient Greek and her Ph.D. in neuroscience from the UCSD. She started her career as a neuroanatomist, specializing in light and electron microscopy, but her main research for the past 15 years focused on informatics for neuroscience (i.e., neuroinformatics). She led the Neuroscience Information Framework (NIF), a national project to establish a uniform resource description framework for neuroscience, and the National Institute of Diabetes and Digestive and Kidney Diseases Information Network (dkNET), a portal for connecting researchers in digestive, kidney, and metabolic disease to data, tools, and materials. She just completed 5 years as editor-in-chief of *Brain and Behavior*, an open access journal, and has just launched a new journal as editor-in-chief, *NeuroCommons*, with BMC. Dr. Martone is past president of FORCE11, an organization dedicated to advancing scholarly communication and e-scholarship. She completed 2 years as the chair of the Council on Training, Science, and Infrastructure for the International Neuroinformatics Coordinating Facility and is now the chair of the Governing Board. Since retiring, she served as the director of biological sciences for Hypothesis, a technology non-profit developing an open annotation layer for the web (2015–2018) and founded SciCrunch, a technology start-up based on technologies developed by NIF and dkNET.

ALEXA McCRAY is professor of medicine at Harvard Medical School and the Department of Medicine, Beth Israel Deaconess Medical Center. She conducts research on knowledge representation and discovery, with a special focus on the significant problems that persist in the curation, dissemination, and exchange of scientific and clinical information in biomedicine and health. Dr. McCray is the former director of the Lister Hill National Center for Biomedical Communications, a research division of the National Library of Medicine at the National Institutes of Health (NIH). While at NIH, she directed the design and development of a number of national information resources, including ClinicalTrials.gov. Before joining NIH, she was on the research staff of IBM's T.J. Watson Research Center. She received a Ph.D. from Georgetown University and for 3 years was on the faculty there. She conducted predoctoral research at MIT. Dr. McCray joined Harvard Medical School in 2005, where she was founding co-director of the Center for Biomedical Informatics and associate director of the Francis A. Countway Library of Medicine. Dr. McCray was elected to the National Academy of Medicine in 2001 and is chair of the National Academies Board on Research Data and Information. She is a fellow of the American Association for the Advancement of Science, a fellow of the American College of Medical Informatics (ACMI), an honorary fellow of the International Medical Informatics Association, and a founding fellow of the International Academy of Health Sciences Informatics. She is a past president of ACMI and a past member of the board of both the American Medical Informatics Association and the International Medical Informatics Association. She is a former editor-in-chief of *Methods of Information in Medicine*, and she is a past member of the editorial board of the *Journal of the American Medical Informatics Association*. She chaired the 2018 National Academies consensus study entitled Open Science by Design: Realizing a Vision for 21st Century Research.

MICHELLE MEYER is an assistant professor and associate director, research ethics, in the Center for Translational Bioethics and Health Care Policy at Geisinger, a large, integrated health system in Pennsylvania and New Jersey, where she chairs the Institutional Review Board (IRB) Leadership Committee and directs the Research Ethics Advice and Consultation Service. She is also faculty codirector of Geisinger's Applied Behavioral Insights Team (a.k.a. "nudge unit") in Geisinger's Steele Institute for Health Innovation. Her empirical and normative research focuses on judgment and decision making by patients, clinicians, research participants, and IRBs that has implications for law, ethics, or policy. She has served on the advisory board of the Social Science Genetic Association Consortium; the board of directors of the Open Humans Foundation (formerly PersonalGenomes.org); the Ethics & Compliance Advisory Board of PatientsLikeMe; the American Psychological Association's Commission on Ethics Processes; the ClinGen Working Group on Complex Diseases; a National Academy of Medicine/Patient-Centered Outcomes Research Institute working group on generating stakeholder support and demand for health data sharing, linkage, and use; and a Defense Advanced Research Projects Agency–funded technical exchange on complex social systems. She developed a commissioned white paper addressing ethical issues raised by plans for developing a new data-sharing institute. In most of those roles, she has focused on consent; data privacy; and data access and use, especially with respect to genomic data. Immediately before joining the faculty at Geisinger, Dr. Meyer was an assistant professor and director of bioethics policy in the Clarkson University–Icahn School of Medicine at Mount Sinai School of Medicine Bioethics Program and adjunct faculty at Albany Law School. Previously, she was an academic fellow at the Petrie-Flom Center for Health Law Policy, Biotechnology, and Bioethics at Harvard Law School, a Greenwall Fellow in Bioethics and Health Policy at The Johns Hopkins and Georgetown Universities, and a research fellow at the John F. Kennedy School of Government at

Harvard. She earned a Ph.D. in religious studies, with a focus on practical ethics, from the University of Virginia under the supervision of James F. Childress and a J.D. from Harvard Law School, where she was an editor of the *Harvard Law Review*. Following law school, she clerked for Judge Stanley Marcus of the U.S. Court of Appeals for the Eleventh Circuit. She graduated summa cum laude from Dartmouth College.

WILLIAM STEAD is chief strategy officer for Vanderbilt University Medical Center (VUMC). In this capacity, he facilitates structured decision making to achieve strategic goals and concept development to nurture system innovation. Dr. Stead received his B.A., M.D., and residency training in internal medicine and nephrology from Duke University. He remained on Duke's faculty in nephrology as the physician in the physician-engineer partnership that developed The Medical Record, one of the first practical electronic medical record systems. He also helped Duke build one of the first patient-centered hospital information systems (IBM's PCS/ADS). He came to VUMC in 1991 and holds appointments as the McKesson Foundation Professor of Biomedical Informatics and Professor of Medicine. For two decades, he guided development of the Department of Biomedical Informatics and operational units providing information infrastructure to support health care, education, and research programs of the Medical Center. He aligned organizational structure, informatics architecture, and change management to bring cutting-edge research in decision support, visualization, natural language processing, data mining, and data privacy into clinical practice. His current focus is on system-based care, learning and research leading toward personalized medicine, and population health management. Dr. Stead is a founding fellow of both the American College of Medical Informatics and the American Institute for Engineering in Biology and Medicine. He served as founding editor-in-chief of the *Journal of the American Medical Informatics Association*. His awards include the Collen Award for Excellence in Medical Informatics and the Lindberg Award for Innovation in Informatics. Most recently, the American Medical Informatics Association named the Award for Thought Leadership in Informatics in his honor. He served as president of the American College of Medical Informatics, chairman of the Board of Regents of the National Library of Medicine, presidential appointee to the Commission on Systemic Interoperability, chair of the National Research Council Committee on Engaging the Computer Science Research Community in Health Care Informatics, and co-chair of the Institute of Medicine Committee on the Recommended Social and Behavioral Domains and Measures for Electronic Health Records. He chairs the National Committee for Vital and Health Statistics of the Department of Health and Human Services and the Technical Advisory Committee of the Center for Medical

Interoperability. He is a member of the Council of the National Academy of Medicine, and the American Medical Association's Journal Oversight Committee. In addition to his academic and advisory responsibilities, Dr. Stead is a director of HealthStream.

LARS VILHUBER is presently on the faculty of the Department of Economics at Cornell University, executive director of the ILR School's Labor Dynamics Institute, a senior research associate at the ILR School at Cornell University, Ithaca, and affiliated with the U.S. Census Bureau (Center for Economic Studies, CES). He holds a Ph.D. in economics from Université de Montréal, Montreal, Canada, having previously studied economics at the Universität Bonn, Germany, and Fernuniversität Hagen, Germany. He has worked in both academic and government research positions and continues to consult and collaborate with government and statistical agencies in Canada, the United States, and Europe. His research interests lie in the dynamics of the labor market: Working with highly detailed longitudinally linked data, he has analyzed the effects and causes of mass layoffs, worker mobility, and the interaction between housing and the local labor market. Over the years, he has also gained extensive expertise on the data needs of economists and other social scientists, having been involved in the creation and maintenance of several data systems designed with analysis, publication, replicability, and maintenance of large-scale code bases in mind. His research in statistical disclosure limitation issues is a direct consequence of his profound interest in making data available in a multitude of formats to the broadest possible audience. His knowledge about various data enclave systems comes from both personal experience and the desire to improve the experience of others. He is data editor of the *American Economic Association* and managing editor of the *Journal of Privacy and Confidentiality*; chair of the Scientific Advisory Committee of the Centre d'accès sécurisé aux données in France and senior advisor of the New York Federal Statistical Research Data Centers in the United States.

C

Registered In-Person Workshop Participants

Ilkay Altintas, San Diego Supercomputer Center, University of California, San Diego
Sameer Antani, National Institutes of Health
Tom Arrison, National Academies of Sciences, Engineering, and Medicine
Nuno Bandeira, University of California, San Diego
Charles Barlow, Cambridge Associates
Partha Bhattacharyya, National Institutes of Health
Philip Bourne, University of Virginia
Patti Brennan, National Library of Medicine, National Institutes of Health
William Bruner, Gadgettronix
Edward Bunker, Johns Hopkins University School of Medicine
Atul Butte, University of California, San Francisco
Linda Casola, National Academies of Sciences, Engineering, and Medicine
John Chodacki, University of California Curation Center, California Digital Library
Sayeed Choudhury, Johns Hopkins University
David Chu, Institute for Defense Analyses
Patricia Cifuentes, independent researcher
Rebecca Clark, National Institutes of Health
Melissa Cragin, San Diego Supercomputer Center
Ivor D'Souza, National Library of Medicine

Maria Doa, U.S. Environmental Protection Agency
Benjamin Falk, Johns Hopkins University
Adam Ferguson, University of California, San Francisco
Jason Gerson, Patient-Centered Outcomes Research Institute
Maëva Ghonda, Institute of Electrical and Electronics Engineers
Jessica Gill, National Institutes of Health
John Glaser, Cerner
Celia Guillen, Johns Hopkins University
Bingqi Han, George Washington University
Ben Heywood, Patients Like Me
Jennifer Hinners, National Academies of Sciences, Engineering, and Medicine
Michelle Holko, Booz Allen Hamilton
Mike Huerta, National Institutes of Health
David Kennedy, University of Massachusetts Medical School
Warren Kibbe, Duke University
Tyler Kloefkorn, National Academies of Sciences, Engineering, and Medicine
Kim Lee, Research Scholar
Young Joo Lee, Johns Hopkins University
Margaret Levenstein, University of Michigan
Tianxiao Li, Yale University
Clifford Lynch, Coalition for Networked Information
Duncan MacCannell, Center for Disease Control and Prevention
Sammantha Magsino, National Academies of Sciences, Engineering, and Medicine
David Maier, Portland State University
Bilal Malik, Kashmir University
Brad Malin, Vanderbilt University Medical Center
Charles Manski, Northwestern University
Maryann Martone, University of California, San Diego
Monica McCormick, University of Delaware Library
Alexa McCray, Harvard Medical School
Michelle Meyer, Center for Translational Bioethics and Health Care Policy, Geisinger
Ilene Mizrachi, National Institutes of Health
Richard Morris, MGI
Oscar Munoz, Algoptimal, LLC
Ron Nakao, Stanford Libraries
Wendy Nilsen, National Science Foundation
Sarah Nusser, Iowa State University
Amy O'Hara, Georgetown University
Lucy Ofiesh, Center for Open Science

Chuba Oraka, University of the Potomac
James Ostell, National Institutes of Health
Trevor Owens, U.S. Library of Congress
Dina Paltoo, National Institutes of Health
Kim Pruitt, National Institutes of Health
Ronald Przygodzki, U.S. Department of Veterans Affairs
Morufu Raimi, Niger Delta University
Rachel Rabbitt, Cambridge Associates
Judy Ruttenberg, Association of Research Libraries
Bob Samors, Association of American Universities/Association of Public and Land-Grant Universities APARD Initiative
Michelle Schwalbe, National Academies of Sciences, Engineering, and Medicine
Shurjo Sen, National Institutes of Health
William Stead, Vanderbilt University Medical Center
James Taylor, Johns Hopkins University
Jessie Tenenbaum, Department of Health and Human Services, North Carolina
Georgia Tourassi, Oak Ridge National Laboratory
Lars Vilhuber, Cornell University
Valerie Virta, National Institutes of Health
Cynthia Hudson Vitale, Pennsylvania State University
ChiLan Vu, Eden Center
Linda Walker, National Academies of Sciences, Engineering, and Medicine
Ellen Wann, National Institutes of Health
Nick Weber, National Institutes of Health
Scott Weidman, National Academies of Sciences, Engineering, and Medicine
Ken Wiley, National Institutes of Health
KJ Wilkins, National Institutes of Health
Robert Williams, University of Tennessee Health Science Center
Tamae Wong, National Institute of Standards and Technology
Yining Xie, GS
Maryam Zaringhalam, National Institutes of Health